THE
RIGHT
DIET

THE RIGHT DIET:

HOW TO CHOOSE IT

BESSIE DITURI, MD, FAAP, FACP

FOREWORD BY SAMUEL GURIN, PhD

NYT Quadrangle/The New York Times Book Co.

Book design: Beth Tondreau

Library of Congress Cataloging in Publication Data

Dituri, Bessie.
  The right diet.

  Bibliography: p.
  Includes index.
  1. Reducing. 2. Reducing diets. 3. Nutrition.
4. Food habits. I. Title. [DNLM: 1. Diet, Reducing.
2. Nutrition—Popular work. WD212 D619h]
RM222.2.D59 1977   613.2′5   76–9700
ISBN 0–8129–0642–X

To the memory of my mother

We might have had the benefit of her wisdom longer had she known the contents of this book when she was young

ACKNOWLEDGMENTS

I would like to express my appreciation to the following people for their help in making this book a reality:

Shana Alexander
Frank Dituri
Fraida Dubin
Emanuel Geltman
Rebecca Herman
Anne Bailey Keller
Terri Korostoff
The research department staff at the Los Angeles County Medical Association Library

CONTENTS

FOREWORD

Many people, by now, have begun to realize that a high standard of living and advanced industrial technology have produced strange and frequently abnormal feeding habits. Prosperity breeds over-eating and elevated body weight; highly refined and processed foods have changed our eating habits; youngsters practically live on junk foods, sweets and soft drinks. As this book indicates, abnormal and sometimes dangerous metabolic alterations can result from current dietary habits.

That treatment of obesity and overweight is an important national problem is attested to by the fact that the weight-control industry cashes in to the tune of at least 10 billion dollars a year. All kinds of dietary gimmicks and weight-reducing gadgets are sold to a gullible public; short term dangerous drugs, hormones and other chemical substances have been exploited in the same way.

The hazards are real; the potential danger to unwary individuals can be great—and Dr. Dituri tells it "like it is." From years of clinical practice and her own experience with dietary problems, she has developed reasonable, practical procedures which go a long way toward solving the primary problem: *After weight loss, how can one maintain it for a lifetime?*

Dr. Dituri's scientific training is impeccable; her clinical experience is extensive. In this book she demonstrates the honesty and integrity that are apparent to all who know her. This volume reflects that sincerity, as well as her very earnest effort to explain the dangers involved, and those dietary and other procedures which can benefit the overweight individual and *maintain that benefit.* The explanations are easy to follow, and the facts are accurate as we understand them today. In sum, the book is a sensible and critical discussion of the over-weight problem by a knowledgeable, experienced and sincere physician. It makes sense.

Samuel Gurin, PH.D.

INTRODUCTION

A new infusion of common sense is long overdue in the weight-control field. Technology has propelled us into outer space, has revolutionized food processing and production in this country and made famine and food shortages things of the past. But technology has not yet made us "bionic" people—people perfected technologically to the point of being immune to physical infirmity.

The metabolism by which our bodies turn food into energy was programmed into our genes millions of years ago—and it hasn't changed. Our ancestors foraged for food, eating roots, grains, seeds, berries and other fruits and nuts, and were able to survive on these lean pickings. Occasionally, meat was available, and our ancestors ate heartily and stored body fat for the lean months that followed. Our bodies retain the same ability to store fat in times of plenty and to use stored fat in times of scarcity, but this cycle has been replaced by a fairly consistent availability of food of all sorts.

The more general problem in our society today is that of overweight. Some of us have inherited from our ancestors certain dangerous genes that "sleep" in our bodies until overweight, eating too much of certain foods, or aging awaken them. Weight problems may be complicated by a medical history of diabetes, hypertension, or coronary disease. The best practice is to employ common sense and to practice preventive measures to keep as fit as possible.

Any conscientious program for weight control must begin with educated common sense. This means not being swayed by tricks and fads promising quick weight loss. Weight is something you have to control all by yourself. Knowing how you eat and why you eat, what you need to eat and how much, and why you want to or should lose weight are all part of the knowledge required for maintaining your ideal weight for a lifetime. In the chapters that follow, you will find conservative medical advice and experience—facts that have been culled from intensive research over the past fifty years. These facts have been a personal guide to solving my own weight problem. The truth is that anyone can lose weight and maintain an ideal weight for a lifetime.

Let me guide you to this new educated common sense about weight control. It can last for the rest of a long and healthy lifetime.

YOU AND YOUR BODY

Understand
Your Appetite

Why Do You Eat?

It's mealtime?
Other people are eating?
Some signal from your stomach?
It's so easy to do?
It's a habit?
Food looks and smells so good?
You don't want to waste food?
You must clean off your plate?

Any or all of these may be your reason, but primarily you eat because *you are hungry.*

Any living creature must eat to survive. What brought you this far through your ancestral chain is *appetite.*

What Is Appetite?

In the earliest stages of life, appetite is instinctive, a reflex behavior. The reflex actions of rooting for food and sucking are present in every healthy newborn of every live-born species. No learning is involved. These reflexes arise in the lower-most portion of the brain; the sense of smell is intimately related to them. Babies root where they smell food. Then they suck it.

But these reflexes, necessary for survival, are soon overlaid with learned behaviors. Babies' appetites differ: Some babies have hearty appetites and can be pressured to eat more and more. Other babies are picky eaters. Some eat every few hours if food is offered. Some vomit excess. Individual appetite differences are as visible in the first days of life as at any other time.

As a baby grows, everything about life becomes more complex. Appetite and hunger become mixed with other feelings. As each day, week, month, and year of life passes, it becomes harder to be sure which eating practices are learned and which come along as instincts. By early childhood, learning and habits have tremendously conditioned the reflex behavior.

What Signals You to Eat?

As yet, medical science has not been able to single out the exact source of appetite and hunger in the body. There are only theories. To be most useful, an explanation of the desire to eat also has to explain the signal to stop eating.

Does an empty stomach cause hunger while a full stomach brings satisfaction? Not always.

Some people report feelings of intense satisfaction from stomach distention. They say they feel full only after eating lots of food. It doesn't matter what the food is. Yet others, whose stomachs have been surgically removed, say they still experience feelings of hunger and satiety even without a stomach. They report hunger and satiety from different tastes, sensations, and foods. For some, small, frequent meals of high-density foods (foods with many calories for their volume) may be most satisfying.

There also are perfectly healthy people who say they rarely feel hungry. They eat out of habit and according to custom, not from inner sensations.

And most of us, no matter how full we may feel, require little enticement to eat more of a favorite food. This is so common it's called the "Thanksgiving syndrome."

As you can see, any explanation based wholly on feelings of hunger or fullness has limitations.

Does a grumbling stomach mean it's time to eat? In a study of hunger and satiety, volunteer adults were hooked to a device that recorded stomach gurgling and rumbling. When the device showed rumbling, the volunteer was asked: "Are you hungry?" Some were and some weren't. There turned out to be little correlation between feelings of hunger and recordings of stomach gurgling. There was even less correlation in the *overweight* volunteers.

It's hard to give up the idea that gurgling means eat. And whether *overreacting* to the rumbling signal is a cause or a result of overweight, or neither, no one can say.

We need to accept the many differences that exist in the ways people eat and feel satisfaction. Common sense tells us that some people have stronger appetite instincts than others. Are these appetite instincts so strong in some of us that the satiety instincts are easily overpowered?

Let's not forget that there are people who can eat a healthy, balanced diet, get sufficient satisfaction, and keep the right weight without giving the matter much thought. Did they inherit this instinct for a balanced diet?

That appetite for food is inherited is a possibility. But not taste; that is learned. We are speaking of large or small appetite and whether a person needs a small or a large amount of food in order to feel full. It is, however, hard to tell whether appetite for food is inherited or acquired.

People from the same family tend to eat together and even if they eventually move to different places, they tend to follow the same style of eating they learned with the family.

You have to understand your own appetite.

Do You Know When You're Hungry?

The chief practical value of knowing a little about appetite and satiety is to establish *self-awareness* of these deep feelings.

When a feeling says *hunger* to you, you could be mistaken. How do we know this? There are factors for regulation of eating behaviors in the brain, blood, and gastrointestinal tract. The brain-appetite-satiety regulator is like a thermostat. The setting, called the *appestat,* varies from person to person. Some are set at sixty-five and some at eighty-two. Or anywhere in between.

Inheritance, learning, habits, body chemistry, and possibly current body weight affect the setting. Some people have a finely tuned set-point that is not very responsive to changes in life style and physical activity. Others have a wavering setting that will change readily with life changes.

Glucose (blood sugar) is the most significant regulator of appetite and fullness. When blood sugar drops too low, you feel hungry and you eat. Blood sugar begins to rise about twenty minutes after you've started to eat. Normally, when blood sugar rises, you feel satisfied.

Do You Know When You're Satisfied?

The signal to stop eating is even harder to define. Studies show that hunger satisfaction from the mouth part of eating—taste, chewing, texture—begins even *before* the blood glucose starts to change.

Few people comment on the satisfying warmth they get from eating. Perhaps we take this sensation for granted. Food imparts a very important heat factor to all of animal life. Hunger has been relieved in laboratory animals by artificially warming their brains. Awareness of this feeling of warmth after a meal has helped people to define better their own sensations of fullness.

Defining and sorting out your own pattern of hunger-fullness serves as a guide to unlearning old, bad habits and learning new, good ones.

What Gets You to the Refrigerator?

Don't beg off by saying you have an abnormal appetite. The number of clear-cut appetite abnormalities is small. But as for hunger, normal variations and the amounts and kinds of foods needed to satisfy it are so broad that we must be careful where we draw the line.

Athletes or workers who spend six hours or more a day in strenuous physical activity eat about 6,000 to 7,000 calories a day. Massively overweight people (those weighing 300 pounds or more) eat about 6,000 to 7,000 calories a day. It is reasonable to say that the overweight person has an appetite abnormality while the athlete or worker is eating to satisfy body requirements.

Another abnormality is turned-off appetite, called *anorexia nervosa.* People with this condition all but stop eating. They have a distorted negative attitude toward food and have in fact reversed their appetites.

A small number of people have insatiable appetites for *non*food. This condition is called *pica.* These people eat clay, dirt, newspaper, or other nonfood, which has no calories. Pica appetite seems very bizarre and is not well understood. Young women who live on small, one-family farms in little Mexican villages tell me they eat small amounts of dirt from time to time to relieve constipation.

Most overweight people don't have these problems. For most of us, appetite factors are tied into a combination of other factors that together cause overweight.

What are some of these factors?

Decreased physical activity. The commonest weight problem is gaining a steady five to ten pounds a year. Decreased physical activity without a decrease in food energy accounts for many of these weight gains. Take those who are committed to athletics in school or who walk a considerable distance on campus and to and from school, or young people who spend a reasonable amount of time at social dancing. Both enjoy more physical activity than they get a few years down the road after becoming tied to adult responsibilities.

Jerry Hobbs, a sheriff in a medium-sized city, has struggled with overweight for twenty-five years. Jerry played competition baseball in high school and college. When he was twenty, he broke a leg and his strenuous ballplaying was abruptly cut off. He spent the next six months walking to classes on crutches. Between the heavy leg cast and the long time it took him just to get around, his activity decreased dramatically. But he never lost his appetite. In six months, he had a weight gain of fifty pounds. He tried one diet after another because life's responsibilities never gave him enough time to go back to playing ball six to eight hours a day.

Today's housework and baby care require less physical energy output than women once expended. If you don't believe this, buy an old-fashioned washboard and scrub diapers on it in a deep sink. Then hang them up on a backyard clothesline—an excellent stretching and bending exercise.

Another common cause of sedentary overweight syndrome is *pregnancy*. The hormones of pregnancy normally increase appetite. And experts on obstetrics and the development of unborn children are coming to believe that calorie needs during pregnancy have been underestimated for the past several decades. Weight must be gained for the baby's growth, for the afterbirth, and for the increased blood volume needed to nourish this growing life.

This extra weight can be lost by nursing, but formula feeding is popular today, and even small weight gains are often retained.

We are also trapped into expending the emotional energy involved in child rearing without much output of physical energy. Physical activity serves a dual purpose. It lets out pent-up nervous steam and burns calories.

A single huge meal. One meal a day, usually eaten in the evening, is often a cause of weight problems. Do you drive yourself through a hectic day of work at home, school, or in the office? The adrenalin you discharge in these moments of tension gets glucose (body sugar) to the brain fast. But this may deplete the supply. After an adrenalized day, food is not only a necessity but a tranquilizer.

In these circumstances, the natural response is to eat too fast and too much. Fast eating masks the fullness feeling that starts about twenty minutes after you begin to eat. In addition, in a person who eats a huge meal once a day, all the processes of digestion and metabolism are so starved by the time that meal is eaten that every bit of food is absorbed and used by the body. An old notion that calories sneak by, unabsorbed, in an over-filled intestine is no longer given credibility.

High-sugar snacks. Are you one of those people who grab frequent high-sucrose snacks? (Sucrose is the chemical name for refined sugar.) Our digestive processes need to do very little work to digest this sugar. Refined sugar is absorbed into the bloodstream all at once. And the body responds by producing insulin. The insulin rapidly drives the blood sugar down. The resultant low blood sugar causes a feeling of hunger in many people. Others experience headaches, stomachaches, giddiness, or muscle cramps. Another high-sugar snack relieves the hunger or unpleasant symptoms. So these high-calorie, high-sugar foods can urge you to eat more. This is *the hypoglycemic effect.*

FOODS THAT URGE YOU TO EAT MORE

Bologna	Cake
Bread and butter, bread and cheese	Donuts
Salami	Soft drinks
Pretzels	Ice cream
Potato chips	Malteds and shakes
Peanuts	Chocolates
Mixed nuts	Cookies
Corn chips	Candy
Snacking crackers	Chocolate-covered nuts
Buttered popcorn	Alcohol, sweetened alcoholic drinks
Peanut butter	Sweetened, milky alcoholic drinks
Chips and dips, fondue	
Highballs	

Each snack of candy, chocolate-coated nuts, ice-cream soda, malted, cake, pie, or cookies contains 400 to 500 calories of food energy. It's easy to eat 1,500 to 2,000 calories a day of just these foods.

Alcoholic beverages act the same way. Those with added sugar give the body 200 or more calories per drink. The result is production of a great deal of insulin.

Nibbling on high-sugar, high-calorie snacks or sipping high-calorie drinks leads to weight gain in anybody who takes in more calories than his or her body burns up. And it leads to diabetes in susceptible people, as you will find on page 12.

Nibbling alone does not cause overweight. Nibbling itself is far from abnormal. Nibbling tests of humans and animals show better blood-glucose regulation, less overproduction of insulin, less overweight, and better ability to perform tasks after many small meals than after one or two big ones.

Primitive peoples nibble on vegetation and berries throughout the day. Wild animals nibble all day without becoming overweight. But they are not sedentary; they are moving about, foraging for food. And they usually are not eating high-sucrose snacks.

But I have also seen wild animals who are massively obese. These are marmots, small rodents who now forage on human food discarded by summer hikers in the California Sierra Nevadas. Everything carried by hikers gets heavier at an altitude of 11,000 to 12,000 feet, where oxygen density is less than half what it is at sea level. At this altitude, people dump their goodies—chocolate, candy-coated nuts, packaged sweets. The marmots' instincts program them to forage and nibble till the food is gone.

Snacking to relieve upset stomach. Many people snack to relieve symptoms of stomach upset caused by undiagnosed gastritis and peptic ulcer. The foods that relieve these symptoms are likely to be high in calories. They are fats and proteins; fruits and vegetables offer no relief. High-protein foods, such as meat and whole milk, also bring large amounts of fat that substantially raise the calorie count. I have seen a number of overweight people who were victims of ulcers and didn't know it. They all lost weight after their ulcer was diagnosed and they were guided to nonfat milk and nonfat or low-fat yogurt and cheeses and were counseled regarding low-fat protein foods.

Night-Eating Syndrome. Most of the people who say that night eating is the cause of their weight problem actually eat one large meal a day. The majority of night-eaters scarcely eat all day.

Instead, they take black coffee or low-calorie drinks till they are so hypoglycemic, irritable, and weak that they eat one continuous meal from dinner to bedtime.

Some people have been able to stop night eating by nibbling on low-calorie, low-density foods (such as sliced up raw vegetables and fruits) during the day. Others have only to eat a reasonable breakfast or lunch to overcome the problem.

A number of people report feeling better and less inclined to the irritability that drives them to night snacking if they exclude sugar from their diet or take only small amounts in tea or coffee a few times a day.

Very strong-minded people report that the ultimate way to stop night eating is to keep no snacks in the house. They tell me they work up to this goal while resorting to fresh fruit or sliced raw vegetables along the way.

Skipping breakfast. This is a habit of many overweight people. Some say they have no appetite in the morning; others say they try to avoid eating whenever possible. The "no appetite" is often due to the night-eating syndrome or versions of it—such as eating one huge meal in the evening.

Whatever the reason, the result is the same—a hypoglycemic effect relieved by eating sugar. Then, of course, the cycle is likely to repeat.

Working on two jobs. Moonlighters are targets for chronic exhaustion. They often resort to fast, high-sugar foods (advertised as "high-energy" foods) because chronic exhaustion leads to a craving for sugar.

Exhaustion produces *stress response.* Stress stimulates the production of adrenalin, and adrenalin pulls out sugar from muscles and the liver. Inevitably, insulin is produced to drive this blood sugar down. As soon as the blood sugar starts to go down, hunger or another of the hypoglycemic symptoms comes on. Soon after the high-sugar snack has let the body replace the glucose that adrenalin pulls from the cells, leftover sugar is made into fat.

After-vacation rebound. This period results in weight that is hard to shed. You have a holiday of a week or more when you swim or bike or play tennis or engage in other sports all day. With all that activity, you eat without the usual restraint. When the fun is over and sedentary life resumed, it's a struggle to turn down your appetite. Often, five to ten pounds are gained in just a few weeks' time. The pounds hang on unless some extraordinary effort is made to lose them.

Habit alone can make the appetite vary. I often see college students who move into rented rooms with meals not included. They eat high-sugar snacks between classes and get caught up in the hypoglycemic rat race without realizing what's happening. Weight gains of twenty to twenty-five pounds are common between the time school starts and the winter break.

I see this same snack-food–hypoglycemia syndrome in people of all ages who have no one to plan and prepare meals for them and have no inclination to plan and prepare food for themselves.

Just growing produces perfectly normal appetite habits. Some youngsters have adolescent and preadolescent growth spurts so explosive that they grow six inches in a year. During this time, they develop huge appetites. When growing is finished, appetite does not subside right away. Strenuous athletics or heavy physical work keeps some of these young men and women from gaining extra pounds. Sedentary young people get trapped in the overweight syndrome before they know what's happening.

Appetite habits can lead to overweight, underweight, or ideal weight, depending on the foods you choose, frequency of eating, body activity, and the heat lost by the body through exercise.

Response to Depression and anxiety. Some life situations trigger nervousness; adrenalin is discharged and drives up the blood sugar. Out comes the insulin to get the blood sugar down. And we have the *stress response.* If high-sugar food is eaten to dull the hunger that stress induces, the hypoglycemic cycle again sets in. You get the urge to eat more.

In time, the brain and adrenal glands learn to respond to weaker and less important stresses. Blood sugar needn't go down very low because the brain has learned to send out hunger signals quickly. The brain can learn to respond as soon as the blood sugar *starts* to go down.

Once you get into the habit of eating in response to various feelings from your body, it takes huge amounts of self-control to turn off and break the habit. It's easier to learn to eat from feelings of irritability, headache, stomach uneasiness, and shakiness than to unlearn eating from these feelings.

You need to know all you can about your own body and your own mind. Become aware of the way your mind behaves when you are in a stressful situation. Recognize how your body reacts to your mind's behavior. If you feel shaky, nervous, or irritable, headachy, or have a funny, sinking sensation in the pit of your stomach when the big and little stresses happen, the chances are you have a sensitive adrenalin response.

How Can You Approach Weight Loss?

First, find out whether you have an ulcer, diabetes, or some other health condition. Diabetes, peptic ulcer, hypertension, atherosclerotic heart disease, and gallbladder disease have close connections with diet and overweight.

Every person with a weight problem has a personal set of causative factors, but food preferences are involved too. Everyone doesn't have a sweet tooth, but high-sugar foods are everywhere. The sugar urges you to eat more; the fat loads you with calories. It takes a strong belief in nutritional facts to turn away from the most available foods when you're hungry.

The more you know about nutrition, diet, and your personal susceptibilities, the better able you will be to make intelligent personal choices. Nutrition information is as significant as calorie information. You need to know your personal calorie, protein, iron, calcium, and potassium needs in order to experience healthy weight loss. You need to know whether you have any food susceptibilities or whether you can eat anything as long as the calories fall short of what you burn. You need to evaluate your physical activity and what exercise does for you. You will learn what the various kinds of foods do to your body in Chapter 9, and how you can live with exercise in Chapter 4. At the start, it is prudent to know whether you have body weaknesses for fat or sugar. The next chapter discusses these and other body weaknesses.

Weight for Your Genes

2

How were you meant to eat? Anybody can get fat from eating too much sugar and fat. But why are some people susceptible to disease from eating these foods?

If you want to be thin and healthy, you can't overlook the fact that many North Americans have genetic weaknesses that show up from both overweight and popular-food habits. If you are one of these, the best way to prevent disease and protect your health is to adopt a lifetime food preference planned to leave your genes quietly down inside your cells where they won't bother you.

No one is immune to overweight. If you are susceptible to genetic disease of fat metabolism, high-fat diets are certainly not for you. If you are susceptible to gout or diabetes, overweight is certainly not healthy for you—nor are high-sugar, high-protein, or high-fat diets. High-protein diets usually turn out to be high-fat diets, as you will find in Chapter 6.

Diabetes

Overweight by itself makes the pancreas produce more insulin. Overweight and a high-sugar diet together make repeated demands on the pancreas for more and more insulin. Insulin causes hunger by driving blood sugar down. People who are diabetes-susceptible because of inheritance, are even more sensitive than others to blood sugar and insulin changes in their bodies. High-insulin diabetes follows months to years of insulin overproduction. And hypoglycemic response to dietary sugar is more common and more glaring in people who are potential diabetics.

Some people inherit resistance to diabetes. They can overwork their pancreas almost endlessly without getting into trouble—at least without getting into diabetes trouble. Yet high-insulin diabetes is getting more and more common in all parts of the world where sugar is eaten in large amounts and where overweight is prevalent.

Ten to 20 percent of North Americans have diabetes. This indicates how well distributed the genes for diabetes are. Abundant rich foods, high in sugar and calories, have caused these inherited traits to surface. Our sedentary life style makes the situation worse by contributing to overweight. As weight is gradually gained, somewhere along the line, the person with a genetic weakness becomes diabetic. Diabetes greatly increases your chances for coronary disease, blindness, kidney disease, hypertension, and stroke.

Primitive peoples couldn't have survived with as much diabetes as we now have. In Egyptian, Greek, and Roman civilizations, as we know from the detailed records kept by physicians of those times, "sweet urine disease" was rare. Today, there are populations who have suddenly changed from primitive to "Western" eating. These people had no overweight and no diabetes until they changed their way of eating.

"Western" eating means consuming foods that are high in fats and sugar. Popular-food habits call for eating every day the kind of foods our ancestors ate only on holidays. In other parts of the world, when the economy goes up and people can afford more rich food, overweight, coronary disease, and diabetes all increase.

Look at the opposite: During the World War II bombings of London, supplies of butter, meat, sugar, cooking oil, and refined flour were very short. Milk went to the children; the richer food went to the soldiers. The folks at home ate mostly what they raised in their victory gardens. What happened? No one starved and there was a dramatic *decrease* of overweight, diabetes, hypertension, coronary disease, gallbladder disease, and stroke.

Coronary Disease

This has become the top-ranked killer in the past twenty-five years. Some of the chief coronary risk factors are overweight and elevated blood cholesterol. These often accompany a genetic weakness for maintaining elevated levels of blood fats.

Hyperlipidemia is the medical word for elevated blood fat. (*Hyper*—elevated; *lipid*—fat; *emia*—blood). Between 1 and 5 percent of North Americans have this inheritance. That's somewhere between two and ten million people. For hundreds of years, these genes have been handed down from generation to generation. And coronary disease, like diabetes, has increased alarmingly in recent years.

Why?

Overweight has never been as common as it is now. And the same kind of eating that causes overweight causes the emergence of hyperlipidemia and diabetes.

This is eating that *overloads the metabolism.* More fat products are poured into the bloodstream than the body can handle. The surest way to overload the metabolism is with a high-fat diet.

What does a high-fat diet do? First, fat provides twice as many calories per given volume of food as do carbohydrates and proteins. In everyday life, sugar often comes along with fat in foods. Rich foods are easiest to gain weight on. And overweight by itself, even without hyperlipidemia, overloads the metabolism and causes elevated levels of cholesterol and triglycerides.

If you want to lower cholesterol and other blood fats, *lose weight.*

The more genetic weakness you have for hyperlipidemia, the more urgent it is to take off extra weight. Your goal should be *10 percent below the weight standard for your age and sex.*

Body fat is called *triglyceride.* Triglyceride is the same in fat cells and in the bloodstream. When there is too much triglyceride in the bloodstream, the blood gets sticky. Although overloaded metabolism from overweight is the most common cause of elevated blood triglyceride, birth control pills and too much alcohol are also factors.

Cholesterol does its harm by settling out of the blood into minute cracks in the otherwise smooth lining of our arteries. This process starts as early as infancy. Every time blood cholesterol is elevated, some of it settles into the tiny cracks. It also builds up on bits of cholesterol that settled into cracks at an earlier time. The process of cholesterol's settling out and building up into plaques goes on gradually as years go by. Low blood cholesterol helps avoid the settling-out process.

Cholesterol plaques jut out into the bloodstream, but they are rarely big enough to stop the flow of blood by themselves. Other things in combination with plaques stop the flow of blood.

Adrenalin—from tension or excitement or hypoglycemia—causes spasm right across from the plaque. The spasm produces constriction, which closes off the blood flow. The result is myocardial infarction or stroke, depending on where the blood stoppage happens.

Sticky blood from elevated triglyceride can cause little blood clots to form on top of a cholesterol plaque. This is another way that blood flow in an artery can get completely cut off.

Inherited overproductive cholesterol metabolism occurs by itself in some people; in other people, it occurs with *overproductive triglyceride metabolism.* These are the most usual forms of hyperlipidemia.

Overweight aggravates both conditions and makes them show up at a younger age. Even temporary overweight from time to time increases the chances for elevated blood cholesterol to settle out and start plaques.

The two factors have to be there at the same time. First, the inheritance, then the overloaded metabolism from eating rich foods and not burning up enough calories, which pressures the genetic susceptibility to surface in the form of disease.

There is evidence that purified sugar in the diet turns directly into triglyceride in people with overproductive triglyceride inheritance. High-insulin diabetes *always* goes along with this inheritance. But you may also inherit a *separate* high-insulin diabetes gene. This should be a double caution.

Aging

Aging, like overweight, increases the pressure on all genetic weaknesses of overloaded metabolism to surface in the form of disease.

The combination of passing years and overweight is enough to cause diabetes and cholesterol and triclyceride disease even in people *without* inherited weaknesses. The combination of inherited weaknesses, aging, and overweight is grim. Ask any insurance agent.

How much inheritance . . .

How much aging . . .

How much overweight . . .

. . . do you have to have before you come down with diabetes, coronary disease, hypertension, or stroke? The answer is plain, but not exact. It depends on *you* and how interested you are in fitting your eating, living, and weight habits to your knowledge of your family history. The more of your relatives and ancestors who had any of these conditions, the more concerned you should be. Do you find diabetes, coronary disease, stroke, overweight, and hypertension on *both* your mother's and father's side? The more of these diseases you find in your family tree, the more determined you should be about weight loss and normal weight maintenance for life. The more of these diseases in your blood relations, the more you should learn to eat to live—with low-density food.

Can your health stand up under overloading of your metabolism? In order to help you answer this question, work out your Personal Genetic Health Score on the following pages.

Your Personal Genetic Health Score is a guide to your reasons for wanting to lose weight. Your score will tell you whether you have health reasons for losing weight and how urgent they are.

Instructions for Using Your Personal Genetic Health Score

1. Fill in each of the boxes. Use a check mark for positives and zero for negatives.
2. Diabetes *adds four check marks wherever present.*
3. Add up your Genetic Score and read results below:

PERSONAL GENETIC HEALTH SCORE

YOUR FATHER'S SIDE OF THE FAMILY	YOUR MOTHER'S SIDE OF THE FAMILY

Father

Mother

Diabetes
Athero and Arteriosclerosis
Coronary Disease
Hypertension
Gallbladder Disease

Grandfather/Grandmother

GF   GM   GF   GM

Diabetes
Athero and Arteriosclerosis
Coronary Disease
Hypertension
Gallbladder Disease

Great Grandfathers
Great Grandmothers

GGF   GGM   GGF   GGM   GGF   GGM   GGF   GGM

Diabetes
Athero and Arteriosclerosis
Coronary Disease
Hypertension
Gallbladder Disease

Each weakness gene on this page counts one-half mark

PATERNAL AUNTS AND UNCLES
(Your father's blood sisters and brothers)

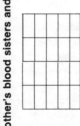

Diabetes
Athero and Arteriosclerosis
Coronary Disease
Hypertension
Gallbladder Disease

(Use the space below to draw in your own boxes if you need more of them.)

PATERNAL GREAT AUNTS AND UNCLES
(Your grandfather's blood sisters and brothers)

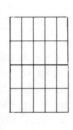

Diabetes
Athero and Arteriosclerosis
Coronary Disease
Hypertension
Gall Bladder Disease

(Use the space below to draw in your own boxes if you need more of them.)

MATERNAL AUNTS AND UNCLES
(Your mother's blood sisters and brothers)

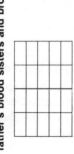

MATERNAL GREAT AUNTS AND UNCLES
(Your grandmother's blood sisters and brothers)

How Does Your Health Stand Up to Overweight?

Six points on each side (a total of twelve or more points after adding both sides) means: To avoid trouble start *now* to reduce overweight and maintain a low normal weight for life.

Four to six points on each side (a total of eight to eleven points after adding both sides) means only slightly less trouble ahead. If you seriously prefer good health to rich food, a commitment to lose weight is imperative.

Four to six points on one side only means that you may or may not have inherited the weakness genes. Look for features such as hair color, eye color, and facial characteristics such as the shape and size of your nose and lips. Very often outside and inside characteristics are inherited together. If your outside characteristics favor the person with weakness genes, the chances are your inside characteristics do too.

Fewer than three points on each side (a total of three to seven points after adding both sides) means that it probably will take a number of years and a lot of overweight to weaken your body.

Fewer than three points on one side only means you probably don't need to lose weight for health reasons.

THE SOURCES OF OUR DIFFERING INHERITANCES

How did our inheritances come about? Geneticists don't know for sure, but here is one explanation that fits the facts: Many generations ago, taking us back hundreds, even thousands, of years, food was scarce and lean. Fats and sugars were hard to come by. People with the most thrifty metabolisms were the ones who survived and had children. A *thrifty metabolism* gets every last bit of energy out of food and stores away every possible leftover calorie in fat cells.

You've heard of "survival of the fittest." Another term for it is "natural selection of inherited traits." When famine or prolonged food shortage struck the land, people with thrifty metabolisms survived. Today, hearty appetites and daily abundance of rich foods are dangerous when combined with genes that were programmed in ancient times for lean supplies.

Living with Thrifty Genes in Modern Times

High-insulin diabetes often goes beneath the surface again after you lose weight. The younger you are when you shed excess pounds that put pressure on your pancreas, the better chance you have of a *grace period* from diabetes. The younger you are when you lose weight, the better your chances of getting cholesterol and triglyceride down, and the better your chances for fewer cholesterol plaques and less sticky blood.

In other words, you have the power to decrease your chances for overweight and diseases of overloaded metabolism. The power is will power— or self-control.

Nearly every day, I see someone who waited too long to lose weight. Remember that aging makes metabolic inheritances stronger and pushes them to the surface.

I recently examined Roy J., a man who has diabetes and gout. Gout is another inherited disease related to overloaded metabolism. Before Roy lost 100 pounds, he was tired all the time, his skin itched and burned, and his knees and feet hurt day and night. His overweight came on gradually over a period of about thirty years. He feels and looks better now; his diabetes and gout are less severe and are easier for him to cope with, but they haven't gone away. If Roy hadn't waited till he was fifty to lose that hundred pounds, his chances for a longer, more complete grace period from unpleasant disease would have been better.

To understand the impact of genetic inheritance, let's look at a province in Finland called North Karelia. There the rate of coronary disease is the highest in the world. The troubles of North Karelia are a good example of how genetic inheritance combined with diet causes disease to surface.

The people of North Karelia are a very stable population; families stay together for generations. The gene pool is naturally selected. The life style is peaceful and free of stress and tension.

The favorite foods are butter and eggs. The national dish is chopped eggs and butter stuffed into shells made of flour and butter. In other words, foods are abundant, very high in density, and also high in cholesterol.

Eating is a favorite pleasure and a frequent spare-time activity. The food and eating styles would quickly cause overweight if the people were sedentary. But overweight is rare because the people work long, hard hours at physical labor.

Yet coronary disease and myocardial infarctions are routine in North Karelian *men in their thirties.* Their genetic inheritance for disease from overloaded fat metabolism is so strong that heavy physical work and lean bodies do not cancel out the genetic pressure.

To see the opposite of the North Karelians, look at the Eskimos, who lived in isolation in the Arctic for many generations. These people are remarkably resistant to disease from overloaded fat metabolism. Their traditional diet was very high-density; they ate 50 percent of their calories as fat. When food was abundant, adult Eskimos ate 6,000 calories a day. They had no diseases from overloaded metabolism.

The secret lies in their genetic inheritance. The traditional Eskimo foods were high in polyunsaturated fat. Seal and whale blubber have to be polyunsaturated or these animals would be stiff and unable to swim in icy waters. Even when Eskimos switch to "Western" diets, high in saturated fats and sugar, they are remarkably free of diabetes, coronary disease, and other diseases of overloaded metabolism. Genetic mixing may soon put an end to this resistance.

Their cholesterol level goes up, but their genetic resistance to overloaded metabolism keeps it from getting high enough to give them trouble.

Roseto, Pennsylvania, also boasts a low rate of coronary disease despite overweight and high-saturated-fat eating habits. The chances are that the residents of Roseto have a much more similar genetic stock than most American town groups. Rosetans appear to have inherited resistance to diseases from overloaded metabolism.

In North America, we have few such stable populations. Most of us move around and mix. So instead of having groups to look at and study, *we have to look at ourselves as individuals.*

You can overload your metabolism with too many calories and prevent yourself from getting overweight by strenuous physical activity. But if you have genes for disease caused by overloaded metabolism, you have no guarantee that your physical activity will protect your health from too much fat and sugar.

You have to control your diet as well. As our country is made up of the greatest mixtures of inheritances in the world, there is no way we can say that any one kind of diet is best for everyone.

Is there an inherited tendency to be overweight? The answer is a blunt no. There is no human inheritance to be overweight, as there is in a special strain of laboratory rats.

Humans can inherit the tendencies for larger or smaller fat pads in particular places. You may have inherited a tendency for fat pads at the insides of your knees, while a friend inherited a tendency for fat pads over the buttocks. But these fat-storage places, or pads, don't show up until you gain the weight to fill them.

Whether you gain this weight is your own decision. The significant inheritance we all receive is the ability to gain weight—and to lose it.

Your Body Outside and Inside

3

Ideal weight is based on height. Frame size too appears to be based on height. Radiologists tell us that width and overall size of bones depend directly on their length. And our bones are, after all, the frame of our body. Independent of height, large, medium or small frame is meaningless.

HOW DO YOU DETERMINE WHETHER YOU ARE OVERWEIGHT?

Standard height and weight tables,* used for years, have serious faults.

These tables derive from insurance-company statistics. Insurance companies realized early in the 1900s that life expectancy decreases as overweight increases. But the height and weight statistics were collected in a haphazard way. Some people were weighed and measured with, and some without, clothes and shoes. Many just guessed at their height and weight.

Only people who bought life insurance contributed statistics to the tables. Until sometime after World War II, many minority peoples were hardly represented. Relatively few women were included. The last thirty years have seen a broader representation, yet the tables still record only people who buy insurance. Even carefully collected statistics do not represent the immense population mix we have in the United States and Canada.

Nor do height and weight always tell the whole story. Muscle weighs more than fat. And there is enormous variation in the amount of muscle and fat from person to person. There also is great variation in body water among individuals. The scale weight shows much more than fat—it includes skin, muscle, organs, bones, fat, and water.

Techniques to measure body fat, muscle, and water separately are available to the research laboratory but are wholly impractical for everyday use.

Skin folds get closer than the scale to measuring fat under the skin (called

*See Appendix, Standard American Heights and Weights, page 188.

subcutaneous fat). But skin folds too have limitations. Many people have asymmetrical fat deposits. You can have a standard amount of fat in the skin under your arm, called the triceps fold,* and two or more times too much fat somewhere else. "Somewhere else" is commonly below the waist.

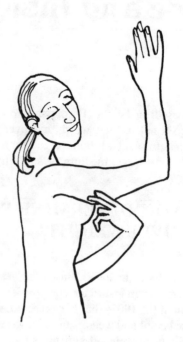

Triceps skin fold

One of the most practical uses of skin folds is to follow your own progress during a weight-loss program. By measuring skin folds in specific places before you begin your program, you have measurements to serve as a standard.

By far the best way for you to decide if you are overweight or underweight is to take a long, hard look in a full-length mirror. You have to be completely nude, and it is wise to have a second movable mirror that will show the buttocks and backs of thighs in the full-length stationary mirror. Look at your stomach, hips, and thighs. Do you see extra bulges and bumps? Do you have flabby places where skin hangs in thick lumps?

Another practical way to establish a weight-loss goal is to get down to the size where you looked and felt your best. For some people, this was

*See Appendix, Standard American Triceps Skin Fold Measurements, page 189.

graduation day or their wedding day. You usually have a picture of yourself taken then to fix your ideal image.

Another realistic goal to head for is a sensible clothing size for your height.

If you believe you have always been heavier than your ideal weight, begin with the standard height and weight tables and skin folds. These general standards, in spite of their faults, will at least give you the range and let you know the direction you're headed in.

THE MUSCLE PART OF THE BODY

As we have seen, the main variables among all of us, other than height, are muscle, fat, and water.

People who spend a major part of their day engaged in strenuous physical activity have a much greater amount of skeletal muscle than the average person. Athletes have very large muscles, and although their bodies look fine in relation to their height, their weight is in excess of the standard tables. Their skin folds, though, are *thin*.

Professional dancers often have large muscles but no fat. Weight lifters and boxers have very large arm, shoulder, and chest muscles. Tennis players who spend a great part of their time at their sport, have considerably larger arm, shoulder, and even leg muscles on the side of their dominant hand.

Skeletal muscles have the specific characteristic of being able to enlarge when called upon repeatedly to do more work. This enlargement is called *hypertrophy*. After growth of the body is completed, physical activity has more influence on muscle size than any other factor.

When you gain weight, your skeletal muscles enlarge because they have to carry and lift increasing amounts of fat. The more sedentary your life style, the less muscle hypertrophy occurs.

Skeletal muscles are jealously guarded by the body. Carefully analyzed and documented medical cases illustrate this. For example, a 315-pound woman who fasted and drank only water for seven weeks lost 155 pounds. At 160 pounds, her weight loss hit a plateau. It seemed that no matter what she did, her weight stayed the same.

The weight that wouldn't budge was *muscle*.

Extra muscle had gradually been acquired to carry around an excess of 155 pounds of fat. A year or more of living with the new lower weight would be needed in order for the excess muscle to atrophy, or reduce in size.

There is enormous variation in the amount of overweight accounted for by hypertrophied muscle in people who look fat in proportion to their height. Muscle hypertrophy also accounts for enormous variation of scale weight in people who appear lean in relation to their height.

The size of skeletal muscles usually decreases with aging. At the same time, the skin folds, which show the amount of fat in the body, generally increase. Standard height and weight tables show that people get heavier with increasing age. But when we get down to the hard facts, this is more likely due to an increasingly sedentary life style than to some specific characteristic of aging itself.

There are plenty of people who work at beating the trend by remaining immensely physically active as the years go by; they retain the larger muscles and leaner skin folds that tables show to be characteristic of younger people.

Unless they are very short, people who are less than twenty to thirty pounds overweight do not have to make extra muscle to carry their weight around. If they change from a sedentary life to an active one, muscle replaces fat.

Muscle helps the body breathe and move around. This breathing and moving around makes a big contribution to physical fitness.

THE FAT PART OF THE BODY

Fat does nothing to help the body breathe and move. But it is an ideal way for freely moving creatures to store energy.

Plants, firmly fixed to earth, store energy in the form of sugar. But fat has twice the energy of sugar—fat has nine calories per gram; sugar has four. For creatures who have to carry their energy supply while they move around, and in doing so burn up more energy, fat is a better way to store energy.

Your body takes food molecules and makes three types of fat out of them: triglyceride (*tri*—three; *glyceride*—glycerin, the basic substance of all fats); lipoprotein (*lipo*—fat; *protein*—meaning that a fat is joined together with a protein); cholesterol (*chole*—solid; *sterol*—a form of alcohol; this is a type of fat that forms into big crystals).

Triglyceride is a liquid at body temperature and is the main form in which fat is stored in fat cells till needed.

When you eat more or less energy than you burn, triglyceride is transported from the liver to the fat cells or from the fat cells to the liver; it rides on the back of special transport molecules, the lipoproteins. Although triglyceride can exist by itself inside of fat or liver cells, when it is transported in the bloodstream, it has to ride on these lipoproteins.

You hear a lot about *lipoproteins;* they are in the bloodstream and are easy to count and study. Too much lipoprotein in the bloodstream indicates that there is too much triglyceride being carried around. It can also indicate that there is too much cholesterol, because cholesterol, when it's in the bloodstream, also has to ride on the back of lipoproteins.

Cholesterol is used by everybody's cells to make cell walls, sex hormones, and bile.

The cholesterol we make in our own body is called *endogenous* (*endo*—inside; *genous*—made or formed). Fatty foods, especially, add to the formation of endogenous cholesterol.

Certain foods are high in ready-made cholesterol. This is called *exogenous* cholesterol (*exo*—outside) to distinguish it from the endogenous cholesterol made by the body. When exogenous cholesterol gets into your bloodstream, it adds onto the endogenous cholesterol. There is no practical way to tell which cholesterol is endogenous and which is exogenous after they mix together in the blood.

All animals make cholesterol for the same hormone and bile uses as the human body. All animal food contains cholesterol. Animal milk also contains cholesterol. Egg yolk and shrimp contain large amounts of cholesterol. See page 214 for a list of the amounts of exogenous cholesterol in foods.

Endogenous cholesterol increases with aging, but people with an inheritance tendency start to make too much in infancy. Progressively increasing weight gain causes nearly everybody to increase production of endogenous cholesterol.

Weight loss, on the other hand, lowers everybody's endogenous cholesterol even though active fat transport is going on in the bloodstream. Exercise, at least temporarily, also lowers everybody's endogenous cholesterol.

How Do Our Bodies Handle Extra Calories?

Triglyceride is always made when there is leftover food energy. Triglyceride is made in the liver and also in the fat cells themselves.

First, the food energy is rapidly changed into glucose (body sugar). Glucose is the fuel our body burns to carry out all its activities.

If you eat a huge high-calorie meal that leaves you with many unused calories of food energy, your liver and all of your fat cells will be busy converting leftover food energy to triglyceride. The more fat cells you have, the more triglyceride you will end up with. Fat cells are not just inert storage closets. Every fat cell is an active triglyceride factory and can make more fat.

If you eat that huge meal only rarely, you might find that you *don't* gain weight from it. Research on infrequent overeating shows this. The excess calories that can't be converted fairly quickly to triglyceride leave the body in the form of heat.

Steady overeating, even relatively small amounts, is much more likely to lead to overweight than infrequent overeating. The body has plenty of time to increase gradually its resources for handling a steady increase of surplus food energy.

How Do Our Bodies Cope with Gradual, Steady Increases of Food Energy?

More fat cells can be made. There are ever so many places where fat cells can be made in addition to beneath the skin: Fat cells can be made in the areas surrounding the heart, stomach and intestinal tract, kidneys, spleen, liver, and pancreas; between the bony frame and the lining of the chest, abdomen, and pelvis. Our bodies can also gradually increase the size of existing fat cells.

Does this mean that humans could reach the proportions of dinosaurs, or are there limits?

One of the most important limitations is insulin production and the condition of the pancreas. Insulin is needed to get the triglyceride in and out of the fat cells and hooked up to lipoprotein in the bloodstream. Insulin is also a must for the liver to burn unneeded fat. As overweight gradually increases, the pancreas has to keep making more and more insulin.

When insulin production breaks down and diabetes sets in, glucose spilled into the urine leads to weight loss. Weight loss sometimes takes place simply as a result of recognizing the disease: the diabetic diet with its calorie, fat, and sugar restrictions, brings weight down. Diabetic complications also account for weight loss.

Another limitation is the fact that each person's heart and lungs can supply blood and oxygen to only so much body and no more. Severe breathlessness is the fate of some overweight people. Another problem is sleepiness because they can't take in enough oxygen to keep their brain alert.

Overloaded metabolism also increases the rapidity of arterial aging, which takes its toll gradually but one day suddenly shows its unfortunate effects.

How Many Fat Cells Do We Have?

There is no way to know for sure. Although one theory says that people who have been overweight from childhood have more and larger fat cells, this has not been proven. The walls of fat cells are very thin—tissue-paper thin. When they are filled with fat, they can be seen under a special microscope. When fat cells are emptied of their fat, they are uncountable. Many of them are used by the body for protein.

Is There Any Kind of Fat That's Harder to Lose Than Ordinary Fat?

There is no doubt that the human body was programmed to cope with feast and famine. Nature has made every effort to provide human bodies with effective energy storage. There is a special type of fat tissue that is more effective than ordinary fat-storage tissue.

This tissue is called *brown fat.*

The triglyceride inside the cells is the same as in all fat. In brown fat, the cells themselves are different. The cell walls are thicker; the nuclei are larger; there are more blood vessels supplying the cells. The cells are more densely packed together. The nuclei in these cells turn out more triglyceride and turn it out faster than ordinary fat cells do. *Brown fat is meant for special survival tasks.*

Human infants have brown fat that disappears after the first few years of life. I suspect that overweight children who were overweight babies didn't lose all their brown fat. Overfeeding and pressing food on children during the toddler stage—an age when it is normal to have a small, picky appetite —is the culprit.

Fat pads that have persisted for years on adults often consist of brown fat. Although brown-fat cells are more densely filled with triglyceride molecules that have been compressed more tightly than in ordinary fat, the triglyceride can still be burned for energy. But brown-fat cells will hold on to their triglyceride stores tightly till the ordinary fat cells have parted with their contents.

This same kind of superfat cell is found in hibernating animals. The black bear, *Ursus americanus,* is a hibernator whose habits and fat cells have been studied in detail. Completely nourished by brown fat gained by summer eating, black bears hibernate for as long as five months. During this time, the animals do not eat, urinate, or defecate. While asleep, pregnant females give birth to young. The cubs suckle on milk made in the mother's mammary glands. The source of this milk is entirely brown fat as the adult bear continues to sleep without eating for another month after the birth of cubs.

Nature gave our fat many ways to perpetuate itself, while modern technology has made the need for human fat storage all but obsolete. For example, protection from cold is a function of fat, but this is of little importance to civilized humans who have devised better ways to keep warm.

Excess fat under the skin decreases the amount of body-heat loss. As fat deposits increase, calorie loss is more difficult.

Nature has also programmed humans with a metabolic factor to make weight loss more difficult by minimizing losses of stored energy.

At about the third week after starting a low-calorie reducing diet, the basal metabolic rate is lowered. This weight plateau has upset many diet plans. You get to the point where the scale doesn't budge. This is characteristic of the fall-off of basal metabolic rate. You burn your food efficiently and on a lower flame.

Various pills and medications have been tried to increase the basal metabolic rate, but as it stands right now, the only safe way to increase the amount of heat loss after a meal is physical exercise.

In the sense that excess fat often occurs from sedentary living, lack of exercise itself perpetuates fat maintenance.

WATER AND THE BODY

There is more water by weight in the human body than living cells and body parts. The body of the average lean adult is 62 to 67 percent water. The average baby is about 82 percent water. As the baby grows, all parts of the body become firmer and the cells are pressed more closely together. In this way, the total body water is gradually decreased to adult amounts.

You can see why water is a big factor on the weighing scale.

Your fastest weight changes are accounted for by water. Water retention or water loss shows up on the scale within a few hours. Up to five pounds of water can be lost in just a few days. Fat loss or addition takes at least several weeks to make a significant change on the scale.

This big, fast drop in weight is encouraging. But water becomes an even bigger factor in weight reduction because there are some unusual kinds of water retention that are characteristic of dieting.

First, *what is special about body water?*

Body water is not pure water or even water like tap water. It is *salt water* —more dilute than ocean salt water. It has a special amount of salt diluted in it. This means that no matter how much salt you eat, your body keeps its salt at the proper dilution—about 0.95 percent. Your body can retain water to dilute any extra salt until you have so much water in your system that you can drown by having it flood your lungs.

Your body is also programmed with a number of ways to conserve salt. Every human being has a hormone produced in the pituitary gland that saves salt for the body. The kidneys do the bidding of the salt-saving hormone to trap salt and prevent its leaving the body.

The amount of salt-saving hormone is increased by stress. The tensions and frustrations so common to dieting and overweight are typical of the stresses that trigger the production of salt-saving hormone in large quantity.

In fact, overproduction of salt-saving hormone may be as common to people who repeatedly try different diets and weight-reduction schemes as increased insulin is to progressive weight increase.

Women have especially strong salt-retention chemistry. The female sex hormone estrogen is a very potent salt-saver. Large amounts of estrogen hormones—normal, natural, and characteristic of pregnancy and nursing —can retain as much as twenty-five pounds of water. Water retention for nursing a baby is not at all abnormal. Any kind of estrogen hormone, such as in birth control pills and menopause hormones, adds to the body's salt- and water-retaining tendencies.

The maximum amount of salt and water retention commonly occurs without puffy ankles and eyelids, though sometimes puffiness and swelling do occur. In any case, whether outward puffiness occurs or not, water retention makes the numbers on the weighing scale look bad.

What Can You Do About Water Retention?

The healthiest way to take care of unwanted body water is to reduce salt in your food. Our bodies were not designed to consume the large quantities of salt that have become part of the food style in the United States. For example, cow's milk contains three times as much salt as human milk. Processed and prepared foods contain many times as much salt as natural foods. Healthy, relatively sedentary people living in temperate climates have done well for years without adding salt to their food. With protection from sun, heat, and wind by sturdy buildings, people need much less salt than they usually eat. Hypertension, a common disease in the United States and Canada, is cleared up in some people by a low-salt diet without other treatment. In fact, *three or four days on a low-salt diet often reduces body water by several pounds.*

But people who are dieting to slim down often take diuretic pills. Diuretic pills, or water pills, work by keeping the kidneys from trapping salt. But body chemistry overcomes this effect, and more salt-saving hormone is produced. After a time, normal kidneys trap the salt anyway.

The result is production of excessive salt-retaining hormone, while at the same time the kidneys are trapping salt in more places than they normally do. People who take water pills for weight loss become resistant to the water-losing effects of the pills.

A diuretic compound is one of the components of most weight-loss pills. In fact, most of the weight-loss medications sold over the counter in North America are some type of water pill.

What Harm Is Done by Diuretic Pills?

In addition to the salt and water effects and the body's way of becoming resistant to diuretics, these pills take potassium out of the body. Potassium is very important to people who lose weight whether or not they take water pills.

There is ample potassium in natural foods. But many overweight people eat mainly highly processed foods that have far too much sodium and not enough potassium. The potassium in natural foods is in proportion to the sodium and acts to protect the body from the effects of too much sodium. Asparagus, bananas, most types of beans, broccoli and corn are high in potassium. (There is a more complete list of high-potassium foods on page 197.)

If you eat between one-half gram and two grams of sodium each day and four-tenths gram of potassium, you are in the range of natural amounts. (One-eighth of a teaspoon is one-half gram.)

But a sodium intake of twenty grams a day is very common in the United States and Canada. When people labor all day in a hot climate, they can lose between five and twenty grams of salt. Most sedentary people rarely lose anywhere near that much. But we eat it anyway because food styles and customs have made us develop a taste for it.

What's more, while large amounts of sodium are added to many prepared and processed foods, potassium is not added. Table salt, sodium chloride, is only one of the many sodium-containing compounds used for flavoring and preservation of food. Look at some others: sodium bicarbonate, sodium nitrate, monosodium glutamate, sodium proprionate, to mention a few. In the meantime, potassium was nearly forgotten until the widespread use of water pills brought its importance to the attention of medical science.

How Do Our Bodies Preserve Potassium?

Potassium, unlike sodium, has only *one* protection from loss by the body. But this one way is so effective that only a few serious illnesses interfere with it. It takes water pills, repeated weight-loss efforts and large excesses of sodium to overcome the body's natural protection of its potassium.

Sodium is an integral part of the body water that bathes the *outsides* of the cells and is a large part of the bloodstream.

Potassium is carefully cloistered *inside* the cells.

This absolute separation of sodium outside the cells and potassium inside the cells is as total and inviolate as anything in nature.

How is potassium lost? In order for nourishing food molecules to get inside our cells, a complex pumping action has to take place. Potassium is a vital element in the chemical pump that operates to keep our cells healthy, nourished, and cleaned of wastes.

Water pills cause abnormal loss of potassium out of the cells each time a molecule of triglyceride comes out. Once potassium leaves the cells, it is subject to rapid loss by the kidneys. The kidneys have no way to hold potassium back.

Chronic potassium loss from taking too many water pills causes tiredness and muscle weakness. The commonest complaint is: "My arms get tired right away when I lift them over my head. I can't reach up to high shelves for more than a second or two." Fat cells and muscle cells in the arms and legs are not the first cells in the body to get scarce potassium.

Cardiac-muscle cells latch onto potassium quickly. This is a good thing. Cardiac-muscle cells must have potassium in order to do their job, and life depends on our heartbeat.

After repeated bouts of weight loss and gain, the potassium losses from the insides of fat cells tire out the pumping action of the cells. And an essential job of the pump is to keep the sodium out in the bloodstream where it belongs. Tired fat-cell pumps tend to let the sodium get inside of the partly empty fat cells.

Many repeating weight losers are bothered by *flab* (also called *cellulite*) —a doughy, soft, cottage-cheesy-appearing skin with numerous orange-peel indentations. What causes it?

Fat cells partly filled with triglyceride, not as yet removed, with tired potassium pumps, have not been able to keep all of the sodium and body water out. When water pills remove potassium, fat-cell pumps get even weaker. When excess sodium and water press at weakened cells with already tired pumps, salt water gets inside. The result is *cellulite.*

Once even small amounts of body water violate the interiors of tired fat cells, it is very difficult to get the water out. The only permanent solution to flab is a long-haul steady program of gradual weight loss via a healthy diet and the addition of temperate, moderate, healthy exercise. The diet and exercise have to be individually suited to the physical needs of your body and to your mental and emotional needs.

What About Salt Substitutes?

Substitutes are one way of getting less salt without giving up saltiness. These products are almost all various potassium salts.* As potassium salt does not taste the same as sodium salt, it is wise to use the substitutes sparingly and to adjust your tastes. Products with equal amounts of sodium and potassium salts mixed together have recently appeared in food markets.

Can You Break the Salt Habit?

The common habit of salting before tasting is unnecessary. Some people who have become aware of this habit in themselves have stopped putting the saltshaker on the table. I suggest a little experiment to prove to yourself that the taste for salt is a habit. Follow a completely natural diet without adding salt for four days. After that, many people no longer notice the absence of salt. In fact, foods such as milk and milk products begin to taste salty. In addition, there are many flavors to enhance the taste of food that don't involve salt at all (see page 165).

It all comes down to this: fat is what you want to lose. Fat loss never begins to show on the scale until after about three weeks of eating less food energy than your body burns. Fat loss shows on the weighing scale only over the long haul. Don't let yourself be fooled by fast water loss or hazard unhealthy changes in the natural sodium and potassium balance in your body.

*Do not use these without your doctor's advice if you have a kidney ailment.

Exercise Is Guaranteed to Burn Off Fat

Don't ever underestimate the value of exercise in a weight-loss program.

The student health departments at two large universities in the western United States—Brigham Young in Utah and the University of Southern California—participated in a joint study on the usefulness of exercise for weight loss and weight maintenance. Results showed that even small changes in calories and exercise could do the trick. For example, if 1,200 calories of food and 200 calories a day of exercise did not lead to weight loss, 1,200 calories of food with 300 calories of exercise turned the tide and resulted in steady, small weight losses.

A number of weight-loss clinics, formerly using mainly a psychological approach, have discovered that exercise is a uniquely healthful way to change the mind from eating to some other activity. Exercise will always burn calories, but it will accomplish the most for you if you enjoy it, look forward to it, and think of it as a lifelong investment for weight loss, lower-weight maintenance, and better all-around health and well-being.

The Low-Activity Trap

It's hard for us to realize how little physical activity we get in our daily lives compared to North Americans in the nineteenth century until we see a jolting example. The experience at Old Sturbridge Village in Massachusetts is one:

The village is an attempt at exact duplication of nineteenth-century America just as Williamsburg, Virginia, is a duplication of Colonial America. Both projects are designed to show how Americans lived in earlier times.

At Sturbridge, they tried to plant and harvest crops with exact reproductions of nineteenth-century equipment. They couldn't do it and had to resort to modern plows and other twentieth-century tools. The Old Sturbridge Village personnel director said: "We underestimated how hard it was and how long it would take."

Nevertheless, many sedentary North Americans today eat nineteenth-century quantities and types of food. Our sedentary life style means we have to replace the physical work of earlier times with exercise.

Importance of Exercise in Weight-Loss Programs

First, exercise burns energy. The human body is no different from other independent life systems on our planet—those not rooted to Mother Earth but free to roam the environment. *All the food energy that enters the body has to be accounted for.* Food energy going in has to equal the energy put out; any leftover energy is stored as fat.

Exercise *always* increases the amount of energy your body puts out. This is true for *all* exercise, even mild types. However, more strenuous exercise increases both the amount of calories burned and the amount of heat your body loses. Both energy and heat losses are increased by activity and decreased by resting. Even when you are eating less food energy than your body needs, the burning of body fat to make up the deficit is increased by exercise.

Body-heat loss after a meal gets rid of extra calories. Physical activity after a meal increases the amount of heat expended from the meal. This is why it's better to eat more food earlier in the day when we are usually more active, than to eat large quantities at night when our bodies are more tired and we are more sedentary.

Exercise does even more for your body than burn calories. When a regular program of reasonably effective physical activities is carried out, it helps your body in a number of ways.

Exercise helps your heart and lungs cope with the stress of sudden demands for increased pumping and breathing.

Exercise decreases the adrenalin response. Active, physically fit people produce less adrenalin. Heart muscle and skeletal muscles also react more smoothly and gradually to adrenalin, so your heart copes better with stress.

Exercise helps your body handle sugar. The hypoglycemic response is decreased. Blood glucose is stored more efficiently and released into the circulation more smoothly. Exercise decreases the amount of insulin diabetics need because it helps glucose metabolism to be more temperate—there is less violent up and down swing of blood glucose.

Exercise helps the heart to help itself. Blood pressure and heart rate are lowered by exercise. Decreasing the adrenalin response and the hypoglycemic response takes stress off the heart. By aiding weight loss, exercise decreases strain that cholesterol and triglyceride put on coronary arteries.

Exercise and weight loss lower blood cholesterol. It is not yet proved that this lowering is sustained or permanent. You have to watch the food you eat as well. The more genetic susceptibility you have to hyperlipidemia, the more helpful it is for you to exercise to keep your weight down. Lowered blood cholesterol decreases the chances of an initial coronary attack and delays the onset of coronary disease.

Exercise and physical fitness definitely make a heart attack milder and decrease the chances of future attacks. Studies are now going on to find out if superexercise, such as running ten or more miles a day, will prevent coronary disease and myocardial infarction. A few studies have come close to showing that it does.

Exercise helps you become physically fit. Most overweight North Americans are not physically fit. This is because so many weight problems in the United States and Canada are the result of a change from active to sedentary life without a cutback of food and calories. You can exercise for both physical fitness and weight loss at the same time if you wish.

Physical fitness is an optimum state of both mind and body. Physical fitness generates a smooth and efficient delivery of oxygen and blood supply to the skeletal muscles, so that vigorous activity for reasonably long periods of time are possible and pleasurable without unpleasant symptoms.

Shortness of breath, pounding chest pain, faintness, dizziness, weakness, and headache following exercise are clues that the heart, lungs, and muscles are not working together in a healthy, effective union. Such symptoms occur when the heart rate has to speed up significantly to deliver enough blood to the skeletal muscles.

A big part of physical fitness is a slower pulse rate all the time. This includes times of adrenalin stress and times of short as well as sustained physical activity. An all-round slower heart rate takes some of the pressure off the heart.

When breathing has to be speeded up during activity and becomes shallow and labored, a person is not physically fit. Slower, deeper, and more efficient breathing gradually comes on with physical fitness.

A physically fit person feels better, sleeps better, and often reports improved digestion and disposition. The main reason these people give for feeling better is that their gnawing hunger pains, irritability, headaches, stomachaches, and faintness are gone. In addition, these symptoms of hypoglycemia bring feelings of insecurity and inadequacy. When hypoglycemic symptoms are coupled with negative feelings about being overweight, self-conscious and easily put down people suffer feelings of defeat. The good riddance of these annoying symptoms brings on as much increased sense of well-being as does loss of weight.

Exercise decreases appetite. Decreasing and doing away with the hypoglycemic response is one of the ways that exercise actually decreases hunger.

An old wives' tale that activity increased appetite made overweight people shun exercise for many years. The theory died hard, but it's wrong and it's gone.

In the first place, doctors who work as consultants for full-time athletes tell us how hard it is to keep them from losing weight. Athletes themselves tell doctors they lose their appetites out of sheer exhaustion on days when they are active for six hours or more. The solution to their weight-loss problem is strictly enforced days of rest.

A controlled study on the influence of physical activity was carried out in a factory. The people in the study were divided into three groups. Each group spent eight weeks in each of three categories. The categories consisted of work at three levels of physical-energy output.

Level one consisted of typing for no more than two hours; the rest of the work day was spent answering the telephone. The work day at level one was five hours long.

At level two, people swept floors, did light dusting, and occasionally filed papers in the office of the factory. Level two people worked a seven-hour day with a one-hour lunch break.

Third-level work was reasonably hard physical labor in the production end of the factory. The machines were old-fashioned, foot-operated treadles and hand-operated cutting, punching, and drilling devices. No power machines were used. Level-three people worked eight hours with a thirty-minute lunch break; overtime of one to three hours was required from two to three times each week.

The results: Level-one people gained weight; level-two people did not change; level-three people lost weight.

In order to make sure that personal eating habits were not more significant than the type of work done, each group of people was eventually shifted to each work level.

The weight results were always the same.

We can conclude that *heavy physical work decreases appetite,* and *very light work somehow increases appetite.* There is more to this perhaps than energy expended. It is probable that boredom increased the inclination to eat at level one. After appetite increased, any number of things kept it going.

Habit, for one, and hypoglycemia from high-sugar snacks leading to increased eating, for another.

HOW MUCH EXERCISE DO YOU NEED?

You will have to accept the reality that weight gains of five to ten pounds a year for five, ten, fifteen, twenty, or more years can't be lost in a week or two of exercising.

Nevertheless, a sound and individualized program will always help supplement a weight-loss diet by increasing the energy loss and heat loss from your body.

If you have only five to twenty pounds to lose, you may be successful with exercise alone, especially if you've been leading a sedentary life style. Still, it's rare to find North Americans with even small weight problems who can't make some changes for the better in the way they eat. These changes are not only in calories and food composition but in frequency and time of day of eating and drinking as well.

Exercise programs have to be individualized for some very good reasons.

First of all, health reasons.

Overly strenuous activity is dangerous for people who have heart disease and don't know it. Even though many cardiologists and exercise physiologists recommend very strenuous exercise for treatment and prevention of coronary disease, people have to *work up to these levels gradually.*

It is far more terrifying to find out about heart disease while exercising than to be told about it at the doctor's office.

A practical way to find out whether you need to have a cardiac checkup before starting an exercise program is to answer these questions:

IS EXERCISE RISKY FOR YOUR HEALTH?

Circle yes or no.

1. Are you a man over thirty to thirty-five years old?   **yes   no**
2. Are you a woman over forty to forty-five years old?   **yes   no**
3. Are you more than twenty pounds overweight?   **yes   no**
4. Have you any blood relatives who've had more than one coronary attack or heart attack before age sixty?   **yes   no**
5. Do you have diabetes, sugar in the urine, high blood sugar? Have you ever had any of these?   **yes   no**

6. Has a doctor ever said you had heart trouble?   **yes   no**
7. Do you have a heart murmur? Have you ever been told you had one?
   yes   no
8. Have you ever had a coronary attack or suspected coronary attack?
   yes   no
9. Do you have angina pectoris?   **yes   no**
10. Have you ever had an abnormal electrocardiogram?   **yes   no**
11. Have you ever had chest pain or a squeezing or pressure sensation
    in the chest which came on during walking, doing physical work,
    exercising, climbing stairs, or during sexual activity?   **yes   no**
12. Have you ever had chest pain or a squeezing pressure sensation while
    walking in the cold wind or from getting a blast of cold air?
    yes   no
13. Have you ever experienced attacks of rapid heart action or palpita-
    tion?   **yes   no**
14. Have you ever taken any drug for your heart such as digitalis or
    nitroglycerin?   **yes   no**
15. Have you ever had high blood pressure?   **yes   no**
16. Have you ever had an elevated blood cholesterol?   **yes   no**
17. Do you smoke more than a pack of cigarettes a day?   **yes   no**
18. Do you have any chronic illness that will put major restrictions on
    the kind of exercise you do? (These include any type of arthritis or
    rheumatism, asthma or emphysema or other lung condition.)
    yes   no
19. Do you have any condition limiting the motion of any part of your
    body that could be aggravated by some types of exercise?   **yes
    no**

A "yes" answer to any of these questions calls for medical advice before
starting an organized exercise program.

The question, "Are you a man over thirty to thirty-five years old?" is first
because coronary plaques are common in North American men over thirty
years of age. Approximately 10 percent of these people have heart disease
and don't know it.

North American men over thirty are close to the top of the list for the
highest coronary-disease rate in the world.

North American women are more resistant to coronary disease until the
menopause. After that time, coronary risks are the same for men and
women.

How to Find Your Exercise Capacity

It is demoralizing to start exercising and then to have stop because you attempted more than you could handle.

Medical and nonmedical evaluations of exercise capacity are most urgently concerned about the heart.

Basically, all that evaluation methods want to find is *how fast your heart rate has to speed up to make it possible for you to perform* a standard activity.

A standard activity is a way of comparing each person's capacity with the capacities of similar people.

Each person who is beginning an exercise program after leading a sedentary life for six months or longer has an individual capacity.

Don't try to compare yourself to a friend. Exercise capacity before conditioning depends on age, health, heredity, and the length of time you led a sedentary life.

Medical stress-testing to study exercise capacity and to try to rule out hidden heart disease can be extremely sophisticated by including electronic measurements of a number of aspects of heart and lung function.

On the other hand, *self-assessment of exercise capacity can be remarkably simple.* For example, try to carry on a conversation while exercising. If you can't do it, the exercise is too rigorous for you.

Jumping rope is another simple exercise-capacity or endurance test. A friend of mine, Harvey Anderson, retired division assistant chief from the Los Angeles Fire Department, tried to get firemen to jump rope for two minutes.

"The firemen laughed at me, till they tried to do it," Anderson told me.

He also told me how he got interested in exercise and physical fitness. "I weighed the men in my division," he said, "and even by using the most liberal weight tables, it turned out that 16 percent were from ten to twenty pounds overweight and 18 percent were from twenty to fifty-five pounds overweight. After one try with the jump rope, most of them were huffing and puffing, and they stopped laughing at me."

Chief Anderson explained that two minutes of jumping rope brings on the same kind of stress that firemen put on their hearts when they first hit a fire and are hooking the hose up to the hydrant.

"The mechanical equipment of the fire department was in better shape than the men, even though we had more money invested in firemen."

Anderson said that the number of fire chiefs who survive to retirement age is very low. He explained that years of tension, sudden starts to maximum exertion, and undergoing the hazards of breathing carbon monoxide, intense heat, and falling walls may not be as bad as the banquet circuits and luncheons the higher-ranking firemen who become chiefs have to live with.

Not only is there a great deal of overweight among the chiefs, but the coronary-attack rate is very high as well.

Harvey Anderson describes himself as the unofficial department chaplain. "When I was an active assistant chief, part of the job was to visit men in the hospitals; sometimes it seemed as if every older, well-trained man in the upper ranks, the ones necessary to think fast and give logical, sound directions in emergencies, was in the hospital suffering from a heart attack. The wife would be sitting by the bed trying to act brave, like in the movies. All I could think," he said, "was that the fire department had lost a good man, the man had lost a good job, the wife and family faced a bleak future. No sooner would I leave the hospital, then I'd be called to another one."

The program for these fire chiefs eventually set up by Harvey Anderson combines weight loss, weight control, and physical fitness.

Just demonstrating endurance tests convinced Anderson of the value of fitness. "After about four weeks of demonstrating, it dawned on me," he said, "that the exercise I was getting while doing the tests along with the men—which I had to do to win over their cooperation—was making me feel better. I felt more rested when I got out of bed in the morning, I could walk faster, climb stairs fast without puffing. It was great."

The retired-fire-chiefs fitness program uses several fitness-endurance tests; one is the Forest Service Fitness-Endurance Test.

A Simple Endurance Test

A simple standardized fitness-endurance test was prepared by the United States Forest Service. Personnel officials at the Forest Service in Montana found that an endurance test was a necessity when too many job applicants and employees couldn't do the heavy work the job required. Building fire lines, chopping wood, climbing poles, and backpacking into wilderness regions are essential Forest Service tasks.

The Forest Service Fitness Test was devised through the cooperative efforts of some of the best exercise-physiology laboratories in the world.

From this combined effort, heartbeat information from the easy-to-do step test was compared with similar data from highly sophisticated treadmill equipment.

The results of this cooperative study were used to develop two simple calculators (see pages 190–191) designed to *predict the fitness level of men and women to do arduous work.* From the simple calculator, you can compare your personal fitness level to standards for your age and sex.

Although the test is not intended as a substitute for a comprehensive medical examination, its simplicity and wide adaptability make it valuable. NASA has found that the test correlates closely with data gathered in more elaborate laboratory settings. The Forest Service and other government and private groups make extensive use of this simple evaluation.

How to Perform the Easy Physical Fitness Evaluation Test

1. Required equipment: a sturdy bench, 15¾ inches high for men and 13 inches high for women.
2. A metronome or some other clearly audible signaling device set for ninety beats a minute.
3. A scale accurate to within two pounds plus or minus. A good bathroom scale will suffice.
4. A stopwatch for accurate timing.
5. Two chairs so the subject can have an initial rest period and for the tester to be able to sit down during the test period.
6. A household fever thermometer to check the subject's temperature in case of any question of fever and illness that will throw off the test.
7. Paper and pencil for recording age, sex, pulse rate, and the Physical Fitness Calculators (see pages 190 and 191).
8. A quiet room with a temperature of 68° to 74° F.

Make sure the subject is at ease and not panicky. Any heavy outer clothing or boots should be removed. Explain the procedure of the test in detail and have the subject ask any questions to allay doubt and apprehension.

Start the metronome clicking before the test so the subject is familiar with the sound.

The test itself consists of putting one foot up on a bench as the metronome ticks, then putting that foot down and the other foot up as the metronome tocks. Each sounding of the metronome calls for one foot to go up or down. At one-minute intervals, the tester announces how many minutes remain before the test is finished. The subject may change the leading foot by marking time for one beat of the metronome at any time during the test.

After exactly five minutes, the subject is asked to sit down and the tester carefully counts the subject's pulse.

Directions for scoring are on the calculators.

Pulse counting is easy after a few encounters have revealed the road-blocks. A good way for beginners to avoid roadblocks is to take the subject's pulse before the test and, with a piece of soft white chalk, mark the spot where it is felt best.

Pretest pulse finding helps beginners avoid most of the errors.

To take a pulse for the final record, start to find it as soon as the subject sits down; then count it for fifteen seconds in order to be comfortable with the procedure. When the preliminary fifteen seconds are over, the next fifteen seconds are the time to take the count for the record.

A person who can't stay in step with the timer because of poor coordination or physical exhaustion must be ordered to stop the test and rest. Poor coordination may be a sign of poor circulation to the brain and should not be taken lightly. Although the fitness test is considered to be safe even for those in relatively poor physical condition, shortness of breath, chest pain, and poor coordination are danger signals.

How do we calculate fitness for people over sixty-five? Simply use the standard for 65-year-olds for all subjects beyond that age. And be sure to congratulate them for having the stamina and the desire to do exercise.

How to Choose an Exercise Program

Once fitness evaluation has been done, the next hurdle is to make wise personal choices from among all the possible activities.

Physical qualifications may be primary, but interests and motivations must also be considered.

Indoor or outdoor work activities are preferred to sports activities by some people who like to spend leisure hours doing something else.

The goal is to choose activities to aid weight loss, and to promote fitness and endurance if possible and if you are up to it.

Be sure your choices will fit your life style, climate, pocketbook, and time schedule.

If your choices don't fit your *reality,* the chances are you'll drop out.

Be sure not to overshoot in the beginning. An activity program beyond physical capabilities and practical application is worse than no program at all. If you have to pant for breath, feel your heart pounding in your head, get cramps and blisters that lay you up for a few days, you'll probably never want to move a muscle again. It's better to build up gradually to more and more strenuous activities than to quit from early discouragement.

Consider boredom when you plan. Unless you are a *loner,* take a clue from other people who prefer companionship with exercise and choose things that fit your physical abilities, tastes, and desires that you can do with friends, family, or a group.

Loneliness and boredom cause as many people to quit exercising as do shortness of breath and muscle cramps.

To enable you to see for yourself what the various types of exercises will do for you, most popular activities are included in the Handy Guide to Exercise. The Guide will tell you which exercises help develop physical fitness and which do not, how many calories you will burn up, and also any important pitfalls and pros and cons.

It is useful and practical to be able to compare recreational exercise and occupational or work exercise. The Guide does this for you.

Here are some important things that cause variations in the calories burned during exercise:

- Individual differences in weight and speed cause variations of energy output.
- Anxiety, high winds, and cold weather increase calorie expenditure.
- Frequent rest pauses decrease calorie output.

HANDY GUIDE TO EXERCISE

All of the activities in the Handy Guide to Exercise are graded from least strenuous to most strenuous in numbers from I to IX.

I. Very low energy output. These activities burn up only a little more energy than sitting and doing nothing, about 2 to 3 calories* per minute or 1.5–2 METS.† No fitness is gained from these unless capacity and endurance are very low.

RECREATIONAL	WORK	PROS	CONS
Isometrics		Easy	These raise blood pressure unless done at the same time as medium or higher energy output‡

*Calorie output depends on body size. Larger people burn more calories and should use the higher of the two numbers. All calorie outputs in this guide are based on a 150 pound person.

†METS means metabolic energy equivalents. This method was developed in order to standardize and classify all physical activities. Energy output in METS is the same for everybody regardless of weight.

‡Isometrics done alone cause the heart to work up against a fixed resistance. If isometrics are done at the same time as an exercise that increases heart rate, then the resistance is relieved and the blood pressure only goes up in very susceptible people.

Isometrics			Hypertensives should avoid these
Muscle-building devices		Easy	These raise blood pressure, not recommended for hypertensives
Strolling		Easy	Pleasant, but very low energy output
Flying Motorcycling Painting (sitting) Cards and games Knitting	Ironing Sewing Polishing furniture Sweeping floor Wheelchair propulsion Auto driving Clerical work Dressing, undressing Machine calculating Leather, metal, wood, stone or clay crafting Power sawing Typesetting Watch repairing		These activities are done either sitting, standing still, or only moving a small amount. More energy is expended when flying or motorcycling in rough weather and other dangerous conditions

II. These activities burn up 3 to 4 calories per minute, 150 to 240 calories per hour, 2 to 3 METS.

RECREATIONAL	WORK	PROS	CONS
Walking, level, 2 miles per hour		The best way for sedentary, overweight people to start exercising	Only one "notch" up from strolling; only promotes fitness in people with very low capacity
Billiards Bowling			Promotes arm-muscle strength but too intermittent to promote fitness
Canoeing, slow; smooth water			Same as billiards and bowling
Bicycling, level, 5 miles per hour		All bicycling is excellent exercise for low back muscles	
Power-cart golf			Not as much exercise if you don't walk much at the hole
Horseback riding, walk			

Playing piano and most musical instruments		Unless you are good and practice daily, piano doesn't involve much muscle activity
Power-boat driving Shuffleboard Skeet shooting		
	Auto repair Bartending Cobbling Janitorial work Radio-TV repair Typing Making beds	
	Wiping floors, light	Stooping causes back strain; kneeling with deep knee bend recommended

III. These activities promote fitness if carried out for at least twenty minutes. They burn up 4 to 5 calories per minute, 240 to 300 calories per hour, 3 to 4 METS.

RECREATIONAL	WORK	PROS	CONS
Archery			One-sided sport, provides most muscle activity for dominant hand and arm
Badminton (social doubles) Bicycling, 6 miles per hour Energetic musician Fly fishing, wading; still water Gardening Horseback riding, sitting to trot			
Golf, pulling cart		May promote fitness if walking is fast enough	
Horseshoe pitching			One-sided sport
Pushing light power mower Small-boat sailing Volleyball, noncompetitive			

Walking, 2½ miles per hour	Good starter toward fitness
Yoga Mild calisthenics	All-weather, indoor or outdoor
Cleaning windows Mopping Bricklaying Machine assembly Plastering Tractor plowing Driving truck Welding	

IV. These activities burn up 5 to 6 calories per minute, 300 to 375 calories per hour, 4 to 5 METS. Many of these promote fitness if done for a long enough time.

RECREATIONAL WORK	PROS	CONS
Badminton, singles	Indoor or outdoor, all-weather	One-sided sport
Bicycling, 8 miles per hour	Dynamic, fitness-promoting exercise	
Dancing, social	Same as above, unless very slow	
Gardening, heavy	Same as above	
Hoeing	Same as above	
Vigorous calisthenics	Fitness-promoting if done longer than 5 to 10 minutes	
Karate	Same as above	
Swimming, 20 yards per minute	One of the best activities for equal efforts of many muscles on both sides of body	Limited by weather, and respiratory inflammations of some people

Activity	Comment	
Table tennis	If vigorous and sustained over 5 to 10 minutes, promotes fitness	Not very beneficial for fitness; too much standing and waiting
Tennis, doubles	Good for skill in tennis playing	
Walking, 3 to 4 miles per hour		
Scrubbing floors, prolonged heavy work, kneeling		
Vacuuming rugs	Shag rugs take a little more energy	
Carpentry, light Horse plowing Paperhanging Painting, masonry		

V. These activities burn up 6 to 7 calories per minute, 350 to 450 calories per hour, 5 to 6 METS.

RECREATIONAL	WORK	PROS	CONS
Bicycling, 10 miles per hour		Dynamic, good for fitness	
Vigorous gymnastics		Same as above	
Jump rope		Dynamic, fitness-promoting, if sustained for over 5–10 minutes; has many supporters; can be done anywhere, complete privacy, very inexpensive	
Horseback riding			
Ice or roller skating		Dynamic, fitness-promoting if done continuously for over 5 to 10 minutes	
Sexual activity		Fitness-promoting if vigorous and longer than five minutes	
Stream fishing, wading in light current		Dynamic, good for fitness	
Walking, 4 to 5 miles per hour		Same as above	
Water skiing			Isometric, except when in the water; not recommended for hypertensives or cardiacs
	Carpentry, heavy		
	Sawing, soft wood		
	Shoveling or digging light earth		

VI. These activities burn up 7 to 8 calories per minute, 420 to 500 calories per hour, 6 to 7 METS.

RECREATIONAL	WORK	PROS	CONS
Badminton, competitive		Dynamic, fitness-promoting if continuous for over 5 to 10 minutes	One-sided sport
Bicycling, 11 miles per hour		Same as above	
Dancing, square, rumba, belly, ballet		Dynamic, fitness-promoting if continuous	
Sexual intercourse			
Skiing, light, downhill		Exhilarating; fitness-promoting only if runs are long	Combination of altitude and cold may be too much for cardiacs; all lifts except chair are isometric
Tennis, singles, includes paddle tennis		Dynamic and fitness-promoting if played with skill so that motion is nearly continuous	One-sided sport
Walking, 5 to 6 miles per hour; this is *fast walking*		Dynamic and fitness-promoting, no undue stress on joints, muscles or tendons; best all-round exercise for most people; its wide popularity is well deserved	
	Hand lawn mowing Shoveling light snow Splitting wood		

VII. These activities burn up 8 to 10 calories per minute, 500 to 600 calories per hour, 7 to 8 METS.

RECREATIONAL	WORK	PROS	CONS
Basketball, social		Dynamic and fitness-promoting if done for 20 minutes or longer	
Canoeing, kayaking, 4 miles per hour		Same as above	
Horseback riding, gallop		Same as above	
Ice hockey		Same as above	
Jogging, a name for slow running, no special techniques		Inexpensive, very popular, easy if fitness level is already pretty good; faster way to calorie loss; done on city sidewalks, or other easily accessible places. Your neighbors will know you are exercising.	Hard on the ankle joints; many people get shin splint; boredom is a problem for some
Bicycling, 12 miles per hour Paddleball, squash		Fitness-promoting if play is sustained for 5 minutes or more at a time	
Skiing, downhill, vigorous			
Swimming, backstroke, 35 yards per minute		Swimming burns up a little more calories than the other activities in the same categories because of body heat loss to the water	

WORK	PROS
Climbing stairs, 27 feet per minute	Excellent fitness conditioner
Digging ditches	Same as above
Sawing hard wood	Same as above
Planing wood	Same as above
Shoveling heavy snow	Same as above
Self-help: ambulation with braces or crutches	

VIII. These activities burn up 10 to 11 calories per minute, 600 to 680 calories per hour, 8 to 9 METS

RECREATIONAL	WORK	PROS	CONS
Basketball, vigorous		Excellent fitness conditioner	
Cycling, 13 miles per hour		Same as above	
Fencing		Same as above	
Handball		Usually actual play is too intermittent for much fitness conditioning	One-sided sport
Running, 5½ miles per hour		Excellent fitness conditioner	
	Shoveling 31 pounds per shovelful		
	Tending furnace		

IX. These activities burn up more than 11 to 12 calories per minute, more than 680 calories per hour, more than 10 METS.

RECREATIONAL	WORK	PROS	CONS
Handball, competitive			One-sided sport; competitive situation; especially in a hot room, is dangerous to anyone not in excellent physical condition
Ski touring, 5+ miles per hour, loose snow			Not recommended unless in top physical condition
Squash, competitive			Same as handball
Running, over 6 miles per hour			

Even though you select an exercise program with care, sometimes untoward aches and pains occur; you will want to know how to deal with these.

You can handle some of them by yourself; others call for a doctor's diagnosis and advice.

EXERCISE SYMPTOMS YOU CAN HANDLE YOURSELF

Charley horse is a muscle cramp that may take place during or right after exercise or be delayed until later in the day. It occurs commonly in bed at night in overweight people who are not in good physical condition.

The cause is being out of condition and lack of exercise.

Remedies are a hot bath, a headache remedy such as aspirin or aspirin substitute, and keeping firm with your weight-loss program. Less strenuous exercise for several weeks is wise.

Side stitch is a sticking sensation under the ribs that occurs only during exercise. This is a muscle spasm in the diaphragm, the large muscle between the stomach and chest.

The cause is being out of condition and unaccustomed to exercise.

The remedy is to sit down and take very deep breaths, and pull your stomach muscles way in. The feeling you want to have when you are breathing in is that you are *pushing your stomach up against your diaphragm.*

Pain in the calf muscles during exercise may be due to overworked, unconditioned muscles.

Try shoes with thicker soles and a more gradual increase of activity level.

This symptom can also be caused by an inadequate cooling down period after heavy exercise. You need to slow down gradually before stopping your daily exercise activity.

If the cramps do not subside, try changing to another exercise, especially if you have been jogging. If pains persist, poor circulation may be the cause, and a visit to the doctor is advisable.

Shin splints are pain in the front or sides of the lower legs. They are caused by inflammation of the tendons that cover the muscles and bones.

Try shoes with thicker soles. If you are jogging, work out on turf instead of paved surface.

Sleep with your feet elevated by putting a pillow or a rolled-up blanket between the frame and mattress at the foot of your bed.

Insomnia instead of more restful sleep occurs if your exercise is too vigorous. The treatment is to cut back to less vigorous exercise for several weeks.

Headache, nausea, or vomiting during exercise can occur if the weather is too hot or if you overdo exercising before you get to the stage of good fitness.

One of these symptoms can also come on if you are not cooling down gradually enough.

The remedies are to wear a hat and minimal, loose clothing in hot weather, and to do a less strenuous exercise or to work out earlier in the morning or in the evening during the hot season of the year.

Prolonged fatigue—being tired even after twenty-four hours—means that the exercise is too strenuous.

Cutting back for a time is the only answer.

Extreme breathlessness lasting more than ten minutes after stopping exercise always means you are pushing your heart and lungs beyond their present capabilities. The remedy is to cut back. If this does not solve the problem, do your exercise with a companion and be sure that you are able to talk, even a few words, during exercise. If this does not work, choose an even less strenuous exercise.

Dizziness and lightheadedness can be due to heat or overexertion.

However, if they persist or recur in spite of cutting back, see your doctor.

The immediate thing to do is sit down or lie down with your head lower than your feet.

Dizziness and lightheadedness along with cold sweat, sudden confusion, incoordination, blueness around the lips or fingernails mean not enough blood is going to your brain.

See your doctor before your next exercise session.

Persistent rapid heart action even five to ten minutes after stopping exercise always calls for cutting back to less vigorous exercise.

If this symptom recurs even after cutting back, see your doctor.

Flare-up of a known arthritic condition.

Use your usual remedies.

Rest till the flare-up subsides.

Some types of arthritis improve with weight loss, and more vigorous exercise can be done at that time.

A change to swimming—easier on joints than tennis or jogging, for example—can help.

Abnormal heart action such as fluttering and jumping in the chest or throat and sudden changes to very slow or sudden rapid bursts of heartbeats call for a doctor's diagnosis before your next exercise session.

These symptoms may be perfectly harmless and the result of being out of condition. Only a good examination will be able to clarify whether the cause is heart trouble or a harmless disorder of rhythm.

Pain or pressure in the middle of the chest, in the left arm, or the throat during or after exercise may or may not be heart pain and should be checked out by a doctor.

Fatigue and muscle weakness can be symptoms of potassium deficiency that shows up while you exercise. When people start an exercise program after being sedentary for six weeks or longer, potassium depletion is common. The remedy for this is to eat foods naturally high in potassium.

How Do You Get Started on Your Own Exercise Program?

Ask yourself if you will open your life to exercise and make it part of your life style. If you will, a good starting point is to take an inventory of your everyday activities (see pages 43–54).

How much physical energy do you put out?

How much time do you spend in an average day doing work or recreational physical activities?

The chances are that when you figure your calorie expenditure from these things, it won't amount to very much. Do you make up for it on weekends by being more physically active?

Is there someone else, your spouse, a friend, or neighbor, who could benefit from more activity along with you?

In addition to a definite, structured exercise program, contributions to both fitness and weight control are made by substituting physical energy for mechanical energy whenever it's practical.

Begin by walking and by thinking of exercise as necessary work.

Walking is still by far the most popular exercise in the United States and Canada. If you walk every chance you get, after ten hours of it you will lose a pound even if it takes a couple of weeks for the full ten hours to total up.

Walk instead of driving or taking public transportation for relatively short distances. Walk up and down stairs instead of taking the elevator or escalator.

If possible, walk or bike to and from work and when shopping, visiting, or running errands. Combining exercise with necessary transportation contributes to your weight-loss fitness program. When you stop at a shopping center, park your car as far away from the store as you can and still carry the groceries.

Think of housework as exercise. Gear your hobbies and social activities toward ways to increase your exercise.

Do you enjoy the outdoors? Consider gardening, hiking, swimming, and walking with other people. Look for clubs that feature these activities in their programs.

Jump rope.

Bike on your own for pleasure, or in a group, or as a family activity.

Jogging is close to walking in popularity. A million North Americans are jogging. It burns more calories than fast walking, and a steady program of at least thirty minutes a day promotes physical fitness and conditioning.

In spite of its popularity and usefulness, jogging has problems. For one thing, it's boring. A well-known cardiologist suggests jogging on country roads and looking at the scenery to overcome boredom. Another suggestion is to repeat over and over a *mantra*—a short phrase. It keeps your mind off boredom and other negative thoughts.

Many people overcome boredom by jogging with a companion. An increasing number of North Americans jog in marathons. The mild competition increases motivation, and the fellowship of other joggers, most of whom are in it for health reasons, is reassuring. It also gives more strength against neighborhood dogs and onlookers.

Indoor activities are available at Ys, gyms, and private clubs. You can find anything from archery to yoga at these places.

Relaxation and pleasure are available from exercise, and it can help you walk away from overweight.

Whatever you do, enjoy it!

To Lose Weight, Use Your Head

5

Using your head is the number one factor in dealing with your weight problem. This doesn't mean that everyone with a weight problem has psychological hang-ups. Psychological problems are just one of the many factors underlying overweight. These factors vary from person to person.

Using your head pertains to everybody. And *self-control,* the ultimate in self-assertion, is the key to using your head.

The more effort you put out to learn self-assertiveness to change eating and exercising behavior, the easier it is to switch your new strength to other problems you meet in life.

If you want to be your own boss, you must have control over your body's food-energy supply and physical-energy output. This means controlling your food and eating habits and physical-activity habits. You can't control your life if you can't control your own body.

If you work hard enough at it, you can get it together. All you need from outside yourself are some directions and a knowledge of the roadblocks involved and how to avoid them.

A misunderstanding of what self-control really is can be the first roadblock.

Self-control is not a mysterious power. It consists of making the wisest personal choices from the nearly endless possibilities in our abundant society.

Some obscure abnormality, such as hypoglycemia, connected with overweight cannot destroy self-control.

Although a condition such as hypoglycemia and its symptoms markedly decrease self-control, in that there is less free choice in deciding what to eat, for example, the deeper meaning of self-control is to gain an understanding of these symptoms and to do something about them. Other than hypoglycemia, there are no obscure abnormalities in 99 percent of overweight problems.

Have You Learned How to Say No?

It is right here that the complexities of life interfere with the instinctive hunger-satisfaction cycle. Your head has to step in and get that confusion straightened out. Self-control is a skill that any motivated person can acquire. It takes in everything from minor changes in life style to adjusting calorie counts for a sedentary life style to overcoming psychological problems connected with eating.

Insecurity is a big roadblock to self-control and mastery of eating and physical-activity habits.

When you can say *no* to the temptations of rich foods, alcoholic beverages, tobacco, and sedentary living, you add immeasurably to your sense of security. This is the same self-possession you need when someone tries to push you around and deprive you of your rights.

When you learn to say *no,* you are started on a new outlook on food and eating. It takes a greater commitment than trying a new crash diet. You are making an investment in lifetime weight control and greater effectiveness in handling *all* problems of your life. An investment in lifetime eating and ideal-weight maintenance is like money in the bank.

One way to get started is to organize your thoughts about why you want to lose weight.

Why Do You Want to Lose Weight?

I suggest you write your reasons down and note the date.

When you write down your reasons for wanting to lose weight, you focus on your innermost feelings. Any self-improvement program will work best for you if you know exactly why you want to do what you do. When your reasons for losing weight overcome your negative habits, self-control is well on its way to making you the master of your fate.

Self-esteem, the ability to get on top of your own life, grows as you find yourself mastering the things you *can* control. It matures still more as you learn to identify the things in life you *can't* control. This maturity helps you make wise decisions about how to cope with overweight.

Insecurity and feelings of inadequacy about inner control are some of the commonest roadblocks to permanent weight loss. Only you can control what kinds of foods and beverages you take in.

Each person's reasons for losing weight are individual; nevertheless, they generally fall into three categories: *vanity, social or family pressure,* and *health.*

Vanity is your inner self, your spirit and desire to be an independent and worthwhile human being. Do you have feelings of loneliness? Do you think that other people dislike you and don't respect you? The more you work at surrendering negative thoughts, the more effective a person you will become. Your ultimate goal is to be more and more effective at controlling your body and your life.

Vanity includes appearance. We live in a society that places very high values on a thin body and how clothes look. But your own personal needs have to guide you to mold society's image into what's best for you.

Close-by pressures of family and friends or weight requirements for a job are the usual *social reasons* for wanting to lose weight. Do you suspect or imagine that other people are making insulting remarks about your weight? Are these things upsetting you to the point of driving you to uncontrollable eating binges? You are far from being alone. If you have been the butt of real insults from other people and can cope with them without resorting to eating binges, you are well on your way to independence.

Do you pressure your children to clean up their plates? Do you pressure guests to eat? Did your parents pressure you to eat? These are all social pressures we encounter.

There are many *health reasons* for wanting to lose weight. One of these could be completely reversible hypoglycemia from too many high-sugar snacks. Sometimes the reason is heart or lung or gallbladder disease, or diabetes or gout. Modern disease prevention always stresses the importance of adopting a life style planned to hold back genetic surfacing of such diseases for as many years as possible.

Are you taking the best care of your body?

Once you have begun to understand your reasons for wanting to lose weight, you have to set your goals. A lifetime way of eating to save your mind, your body, and your pocketbook is the only way to success. You have to take your food tastes, food knowledge, and calorie sense with you everywhere you go. You have to learn the answers to the following questions: What makes you hungry? What makes you full? What foods are good for *your* body? What foods are bad for *your* health? And you have to learn how to make a rapid calorie count of any food in a restaurant, a market, or in your own or someone else's home, and how to say "No, thank you," so graciously that other people envy you your power.

Plan how you will handle all your contacts with food as carefully as you would plan a vacation trip.

When and Where Do You Have Your Problems?

Is your weakness eating candy at the movies or frequent trips to the vending machine at work or at school? Many people have overcome these problems by taking along low-calorie snacks. Carrot sticks are slightly sweet, offer plenty of chewing satisfaction, and keep well in a plastic bag inside a purse or desk drawer or locker.

Are you addicted to carbonation? High-calorie soft drinks are terrible for your teeth and your diet. And low-calorie soft drinks only cater to your sweet tooth and are no solution to thirst. Teach yourself to drink water. When you can successfully cut out all sweeteners in your water, you will be close to self-mastery.

Does your mouth water when you pass high-calorie foods in the supermarket? Impulse buying (and eating) of ready-to-eat high-density foods accounts for much overweight. Don't go shopping when you're hungry; shop with a list based on your daily or weekly food plan; plan menus ahead and stick to them.

Do you nibble while cooking? Nibbling can be a natural, healthy act. Plan to have low-calorie nibbles on hand to eat while you cook. Any of the raw vegetables listed on page 205 are fine snacks.

Are restaurants, especially fast-food, limited-menu restaurants, a traumatic experience? Choose prudently from the menu on the basis of your calorie and nutrition knowledge. Steer your friends toward a place with a salad bar.

Nighttime eating is a thorn in many people's hides. The struggle against this tormentor is hard because its victims are tired and drained of self-control. The other dangerous aspect is that its victims are not really hungry.

Turning off the TV and turning in for an early bedtime is one solution, as nighttime eating is often a symptom of unrecognized sleepiness. A walk after dinner helps many people who fear insomnia if they go to bed too early.

Remember—you fight sleep when you are overtired.

Switching to low-density, raw-vegetable snacks or something that takes a long time to eat, like sunflower seeds in the shell, is another way to cope with overeating at night.

Be Conscious of Everything You Do with Food and Eating

Here you can be innovative. You are the person most able to probe for the cause of your bad food habits. Each human being has a unique set of personal factors.

The ability to control eating of the most tempting foods is a crucial step. If you have gained weight because of hypoglycemia or a sedentary way of life, the foods that urge you to eat more have probably been a source of trouble.

• The only way to kick the sugar and hypoglycemia cycle is to avoid sugar. Substituting noncaloric sweeteners helps, but your final weight result will depend on how many calories your foods contain.

For example, cookies or chocolates contain many fat calories even if they are artificially sweetened. Natural fruits as substitutes contain less sugar and calories in relation to volume. Fruit volume is highly expanded by water and pulp. Raw vegetable snacks are, of course, lowest in calories, as they are largely water and pulp with very little available sugar.

• Learning calorie values and nutritional contents of foods is a big help. Read labels on processed foods.

• Portion sizes are the nemesis for some people; learning to estimate them in relation to calorie count is a valuable tool. The Break the Rules Calorie Counter on page 222 shows you the small volumes of popular high density foods that provide 200 calories.

Portion sizes are important with high-density, low-volume foods. Serving each plate in the kitchen, restaurant style, instead of putting bowls on the table, family style, is one solution. Switching to lower-density higher-volume foods is another. If your choice is smaller portions of high-density foods, use smaller plates to serve your meals on.

• Do you need lots of food? Use your will power to switch your favorite foods from high-density to low-density foods. Low-density lifetime eating is a way to be full but not fat. Many people with weight problems never get anywhere in their weight-losing programs until they realize that they have large appetites satisfied with large volumes of food.

Large volumes of high-density foods quickly add up to 3,000 to 4,000 and more calories a day. Only people doing heavy, sustained physical labor for most of the day can eat so many calories without steadily gaining weight.

Self-assertiveness works here. Assert yourself now to stop eating foods that urge you to eat more (see page 8).

People who have developed a longtime commitment, about a year or longer, to low-density, high-volume eating find the rich stuff loses its appeal.

At that point, you can concentrate all your self-esteem on other things in life.

• Do you think life will lose some of its zest if you stop eating most of the tempting foods or at least cut back to eating them only on holidays or special occasions? *Not at all,* say people who have successfully kicked the habit. The pleasure sensation of feeling full becomes more important than what food you eat. Your tastes change and other foods become more appealing. This takes time, usually as long as a year or more. Don't expect the change to come overnight. Holidays and special occasions revive an old-fashioned festival spirit if high-calorie, high-density foods appear only on these days.

• Do you have the strength to stand up to advertising pressures? You don't have to go hungry because you have tuned out propaganda about high-calorie foods. We are constantly attacked by this pressure, but there are plenty of other foods we can eat.

Can You Separate Food and Eating?

There are valuable lessons to be learned from the ability to separate food from eating. Some people have problems with eating itself.

Do you find yourself eating so fast that your fullness sensation is masked? There is, as we have seen, a delay of about twenty minutes between the time you've eaten enough food and the time you begin to feel full. If you continue to eat during this lag period, you can easily eat too many calories.

Fast eating becomes a habit, and the message center in your brain gets confused about the fullness feeling. Fast eating can be unlearned. This calls for being methodical:

Start every meal with a glass of water. Drinking water helps slow your pace before you start on food. Water starts to fill you up before the food gets to your stomach. It also helps prevent constipation and keeps your kidneys flushed out.

Count bites. This is another way to slow down eating. About seventy-five years ago, an eating fad called Fletcherization took North America by storm. An American, Horace Fletcher, and an Englishman, Lord Gladstone, started the movement because they believed digestion and dental health would improve if people chewed each mouthful thirty-two times. The number thirty-two was chosen because that is the number of teeth in the mouth.

Faithful followers of Fletcherization lost weight. They felt full and satisfied long before their food was eaten up and they left food on their plates.

Relax while eating more slowly. This helps the fullness message get through. Make a conscious effort to put down your fork every few bites, drink some water, and relax.

Soft music, candlelight, beautiful table settings, flowers, and company are some things that create an atmosphere of relaxation at mealtime. Several people have told me that they accomplished miracles in slower eating by planning topics ahead of time for pleasant and distracting mealtime conversation. The conversation becomes more important than the food.

Do you have problems when you eat alone? Plan every morsel and calorie ahead of time. Never eat directly from the refrigerator or cupboard. This is the easiest way to overeat and mask the fullness feeling. Instead, set all your foods on plates. Read a book while eating. Always sip water between bites.

Experiment with different foods to discover how they satisfy you. If you have a dislike for low-density, high-volume foods, work to change your habits. Perhaps you'll find that chewing crispy raw vegetables can be a sensuous experience. Many people have made pleasant taste discoveries by using herbs and spices to flavor vegetables they once thought were flat and flavorless (see page 165).

Write down your thoughts. Assess your feelings and motives for overeating and eating the wrong foods. When you keep a record for yourself of your mental exploration for personal causes and solutions for overweight, you become your own boss. Each memory of a bad habit is a useful clue to your plan for forming new habits.

Overeating and wrong-food eating are destructive to your ego and self-esteem because you failed to have power over your mouth.

But don't waste emotional energy feeling guilty. Challenge yourself, instead, to hold more firmly to your vows in the future.

The records and notes you keep about these explorations are more valuable if you add remarks and descriptions about weak moments. Be sure to record your good experiences too.

Self-discovery notes about hunger feelings, food and eating notions, and so on, have unlocked the secret reasons for overeating and wrong-food eating for many people. After all, you are the one who has to make the choices and say no. And the more information you have about yourself, the better you will be able to cope successfully with temptation.

Keep in mind that while it is fine to get help and support from other people, the goal is mature independence. You need independence so strong that you can face any food or eating situation with total ability to make cool-headed, wise personal choices.

In fact, a good self-improvement exercise is to think yourself into a number of food and eating situations and imagine or develop your solutions.

Think of social situations. Picture loaded buffets, hostesses passing rich hors d'oeuvres and desserts, alcoholic beverages. When you can say *No, thank you* without an inner feeling of having lost out on something, you are liberated.

When you pass up vending machines and other easily accessible high-density, low-volume foods, you are a free person.

When you can watch the endless parade of food ads on TV and not feel hunger or desire to eat, you are your own boss.

Diaries of food, exercise, and eating with remarks and space for daily and weekly totals have an important place in this self-help program. Use the diary on the following pages to get started.

How long does it pay to keep a diary? As long as it helps you unlearn old bad habits and make new good ones. I have seen people who were independent at the end of one month; it has taken others more than a year.

See how strong your self-assertiveness and will power are at the end of one month of keeping your diary.

Reinforcements

Any number of mind strengtheners are available to you. The words and the methods differ, but the basics are similar. Here are some of them:

- *Prayer*—fervently asking a Higher Power for the strength to attain your important goal.
- *Yoga and Zen*—fervently setting the mind to have greater and greater control over the body.
- *Transcendental meditation* (TM) or other meditation—to help you with your relaxation and mind-strengthening by increasing your ability to bear pain, hunger, fear, and frustration. Meditation does this by releasing your mind from its daily burdens.
- *A mantra*—a mind releaser—a key phrase repeated over and over to keep the mind from wandering during meditation.

All these are actually ways to self-hypnosis. Hypnosis is nothing more than an effort to relax the mind and free it from the day-to-day worries and hang-ups, to untie the knots pressing and twisting the mind into bad ways of directing the body.

All the methods rely on concentration, clarity, and objectivity.

As the mind releasers little by little cleanse and unburden your spirit, your body becomes better able to accept new positive affirmations. You become better at asserting yourself.

Part of the basic method of all kinds of self-hypnosis is a push-the-button concept of cue words. Pushing the button immediately sets your mind onto

MY FOOD AND PHYSICAL ACTIVITY DIARY

WEEK 1	Day 1 Date	Day 2 Date	Day 3 Date	Day 4 Date
Breakfast Food	Calories In			
Lunch Food	Calories In			
Dinner Food	Calories In			
Snacks	Calories In			
Water				
Exercise Time Spent	Calories Out			
Daily Calories In				
Daily Calories Out				
Daily Deficit				

(Put this number on your balance sheet, page 74.)

68

	Day 5 Date____	Day 6 Date____	Day 7 Date____	Day 8 Date____
Breakfast Food	Calories In			
Lunch Food	Calories In			
Dinner Food	Calories In			
Snacks	Calories In			
Water				
Exercise Time Spent	Calories Out			

Daily Calories In____
Daily Calories Out____
Daily Deficit____

(Put this number on your balance sheet, page 74.)

WEEK 2	Day 9 Date ____	Day 10 Date ____	Day 11 Date ____	Day 12 Date ____
Breakfast Food	Calories In			
Lunch Food	Calories In			
Dinner Food	Calories In			
Snacks	Calories In			
Water				
Exercise Time Spent	Calories Out			

Daily Calories In ____
Daily Calories Out ____
Daily Deficit ____

(Put this number on your balance sheet, page 74.)

70

	Day 13 Date_____	Day 14 Date_____	Day 15 Date_____	Day 16 Date_____
Breakfast Food	Calories In			
Lunch Food	Calories In			
Dinner Food	Calories In			
Snacks	Calories In			
Water				
Exercise Time Spent	Calories Out			

Daily Calories In_____
Daily Calories Out_____
Daily Deficit_____
(Put this number on your balance sheet, page 74.)

WEEK 3	Day 17 Date____	Day 18 Date____	Day 19 Date____	Day 20 Date____
Breakfast Food	Calories In			
Lunch Food	Calories In			
Dinner Food	Calories In			
Snacks	Calories In			
Water				
Exercise Time Spent	Calories Out			

Daily Calories In____

Daily Calories Out____

Daily Deficit____

(Put this number on your balance sheet, page 74.)

WEEK 4	Day 21 Date____	Day 22 Date____	Day 23 Date____	Day 24 Date____
Breakfast Food	Calories In			
Lunch Food	Calories In			
Dinner Food	Calories In			
Snacks	Calories In			
Water				
Exercise Time Spent	Calories Out			

Daily Calories In ____
Daily Calories Out ____
Daily Deficit ____
(Put this number on your balance sheet, page 74.)

	Day 25 Date____	Day 26 Date____	Day 27 Date____	Day 28 Date____
Breakfast Food	Calories In			
Lunch Food	Calories In			
Dinner Food	Calories In			
Snacks	Calories In			
Water				
Exercise Time Spent	Calories Out			

Daily Calories In_____
Daily Calories Out_____
Daily Deficit_____

(Put this number on your balance sheet, page 74.)

74

MY NOTES AND SUMMARY SHEET

Week 1

Calorie Deficit		My Weight My Skin Fold Measurement	Comments (about good and bad things)
	Day 1		
	2		
	3		
	4		
	5		
	6		
	7		

Week 2

Calorie Deficit		My Weight My Skin Fold Measurement	Comments
	Day 1		
	2		
	3		
	4		
	5		
	6		
	7		

Week 3

Calorie Deficit		My Weight My Skin Fold Measurement	Comments
	Day 1		
	2		
	3		
	4		
	5		
	6		
	7		

Week 4

Calorie Deficit		My Weight My Skin Fold Measurement	Comments
	Day 1		
	2		
	3		
	4		
	5		
	6		
	7		

My Weekly Calorie Requirement _____
My Weekly Calorie Deficit _____

For every deficit of 3,500 calories, you will lose a pound of fat.
Do not be fooled by the scale. See Chapter 3.

the objective you're working toward. Your mind's response is: I will be strong. I will be strong. I will stop eating. Or whatever your key words have been.

Your chosen method of self-hypnosis is the cue or trigger to get your body to do what you've been trying to teach it to do. Make a tape recording of your own voice saying: "I will stop eating the wrong food." Or: "I will stop eating when I'm not hungry."

Tape your voice saying your prayer or your mantra. It is very effective to hear your own voice coming back to you. Your own voice saying your own words in your own way is a stronger, more personal reinforcement than hearing someone else say these things.

Visual imagery, self-suggestion with mental pictures, helps some people as much as verbal ideas. Visualize yourself in beautiful clothes several sizes smaller than you now wear. Imagine yourself playing a sport you'd like to try or going somewhere you'd like to go and being several sizes smaller.

Practice bringing up these mental images at moments when your old bad habits seem to be getting the upper hand . . . when you feel like eating at night . . . when boredom, frustration or anger lead you toward the candy or soft-drink machine.

To aid your mental image, cut out a picture of someone whose body you admire from a magazine. Take a photo of yourself, cut out your face and head and paste it over the head of the person in the picture. Now you have a picture to reinforce your mental image of what you would like to look like. Paste this picture on the refrigerator door.

Do You Eat for Nonhunger Reasons?

You've been in the habit of eating when you think you're hungry even though you know you really aren't. Your habit tells you to eat because you are used to responding to a particular sensation by eating. What nonhunger sensation drives you to eat?

For example, you've just had an argument, you're angry, you head for the refrigerator. Set up a mind-picture method to battle against this bad habit.

Sit right down and force your mind to think of *you* in that new, smaller outfit you'd like to wear. Keep doing this until the anger-hungry sensation passes.

When you've successfully fought off that sensation, write a comment on your Summary Sheet (page 74).

The more often you do this and the more times you are successful, the easier it becomes for your mind and new independent will power to win.

After a while, your will begins to unlearn the old bad habit.

Some people call this process *learning* and others call it *conditioning*. In fact, it's mind over matter—another way of saying *self-control.*

Self-control is getting your body to do what your head has decided it should do.

When you have uncontrollable nonhunger urges to eat, your goal of a thin body becomes hazy and you experience the confusion and cynicism of past failures and backsliding.

Before you dismiss your unreal hunger problem as insurmountable, be sure it isn't caused or being magnified and prodded along by sugar-induced hypoglycemia.

Remember that the chief causes of unreal hunger are stress, anger, fear, and frustration. These can be produced by the adrenalin-hypoglycemia response. Can you reverse your next unreal hunger pangs from the adrenalin-hypoglycemia response by doing some physical activity?

A punching bag is a pretty good anger reliever. Work out on your own so that you take all of your anger out on the punching bag. You'll find that punching a bag will work off your extra adrenalin and satisfy your nonhunger pangs.

Nonhunger eating is commonest in certain stressful situations. Among the worst of these are situations of emotional upheaval and conflict. Runners-up are periods of increased responsibility. Include in this category the times you are engaged in work that makes maximum demands on your concentration or creative faculties.

HOW TO AVOID FAILURE

You have already made huge strides when you learn to recognize nonhungry hunger. Nevertheless, viewing your weight problem as an all-or-nothing matter is the cause of many failures.

You may not be able to redirect nonhungry hunger into some other feeling or way of acting every time it comes on.

Reacting to stress, anger, fear, frustration or loneliness by eating is less of a problem than reacting by drinking, taking drugs, having a nervous breakdown, or committing suicide.

What to do?

The answer is *eat.*

But use your head. Eat raw vegetables and plain fruits without added sugar, syrup, or cream. Fix a huge bowl of carrot sticks, cauliflowerets, radishes, and celery sticks cut into finger-picking tasty pieces; add thin slices of cantaloupe and pieces of grapefruit.

Have a using-your-head eating binge.

Chew and eat to your heart's content. Eating is not a sin and it's not antisocial, as are some of the more dangerous alternatives to eating. The fiber from this binge is *good* for constipation. The vitamins and minerals from this binge are *good* for you. Remember to drink water with this binge; it's *good* for you, too.

Relax in the knowledge that it's perfectly possible to eat without getting fat or tempting inherited-disease tendencies to surface.

Determine What You Need to Do to Reach Your Goal

Whatever means you choose to reach your desired goal of lifetime weight control, your head has to be at the helm and be the boss of your body.

• Your means can be a major change in food selection, only a minor change in portion sizes, or cutting off of snacks that were making you hypoglycemic.

• Your means can be a change from fast to slow eating, from impulse fast-food or vending-machine eating to bringing a low-calorie lunch from home or putting a stationary bike in front of the TV and substituting a little cycling for night eating.

• Your means can be exchanging a few hundred burned-up calories from walking thirty minutes after work for a couple hundred calories of alcoholic drinks.

The means you use are up to you. What matters is that only you can follow through with the selected means to the desired end. You don't have to have the will of a saint or feel that you can never fall off the wagon or go astray. It doesn't matter whether your doctor guides you on food and exercise choices or whether you are in a position to make all your own choices.

• You do have to have a good strong idea of why you want to lose weight.
• You have to focus on the things that are causing you to gain or not lose or to regain what you've lost.
• You have to have strong ideas of how to go about setting a reachable goal and reaching it.

Remember, you cannot *will* your body to lose weight. You can only will your body to take in fewer calories of food energy than it burns up.

When you know what you are doing and why, your self-esteem will immediately increase. Whatever you choose to do at that point to reinforce your will power will simply put you further ahead in your quest for self-mastery. However, some very agonizing fears and dilemmas can create roadblocks along the way, and it takes an awful lot of headwork to get around them.

Eliminate Roadblocks

Fears of failure are the biggest roadblocks. These can come out in the form of fears of binge-eating or fears of having the apple cart upset by life's conflicts and emotional upsets. What to do?

Former compulsive eaters and binge eaters get their self-assessment diary out of the drawer. What does your diary have to say about your causes for overweight or failures to maintain losses or both?

Which of these common causes for compulsive and binge eating do you find in your diary? Boredom? Tension? Self-pity? Guilt feelings over failing? Jealousy? Anger? Fear?

If you are *bored* with your work, you may be bored if you change work. Have you considered a hobby such as painting, ceramics, or needlepoint to use your hands and to channel your creative energy in a disciplined way? These activities leave your hands too messy or too busy for you to eat when you aren't really hungry. Challenge yourself to come up with other ideas.

Tension? Remember how exercise can help put a stop to the adrenalin-hypoglycemia cycle? Explore your life style for sources of tension. Do you have better and worse days? What distinguishes them? What can you do to have more *better* days? Does skipping meals cause tension and later compulsive or binge eating? Try the ways to stop hypoglycemic reactions.

Are you the victim of *self-pity?* The I-don't-care-any-more and Nobody-loves-me hang-ups are signs of selfishness. Rather than self-esteem, self-pity means weakness and dependence. Before giving in, have you tried giving some spare time to people who have it far worse than you do? Helping people is a creative experience. If you can get yourself to do *one thing* to reverse an attack of self-pity, you are on the road to recovery.

Guilt feelings over failing? This is another form of self-pity. Here it is specifically directed at one or more eating situations. It may arise out of moodiness or some other person's innocent but stupid remark. A very useful antidote to guilt feelings and self-pity caused by backsliding is essay writing.

Sit down and describe in writing every emotion you felt from the time you were driven to go on your binge to the end result—guilt feelings.

When your self-esteem needs more bolstering than you can give yourself and all efforts at self-help flounder, I urge you to make outside contacts.

Groups of people with similar weight problems and goals are excellent outside contacts.

Get together with a friend or two and start your own weight-concerned group. Don't isolate yourself. Other people have similar problems and doubts. We each have our weak points and strong points. Start a help-line with one or two friends who have the same problem. Agree to be able to call each other twenty-four hours a day if all other aids to continued will power fail.

Get your group together for meetings on a regular basis. Choose topics and report on them—for example, mind-reinforcing, nutrition, low-density recipes, or whatever areas your own creative energy directs you to. In time, you will be able to interest professional speakers to address your group occasionally.

Or join an existing group in your community. These groups have already helped thousands of men and women.

It is my observation that voluntary groups such as TOPS and Overeaters Anonymous have higher success rates than the commercial dieting enterprises.

TOPS—Take Off Pounds Sensibly—has been around for over thirty years. Members are rewarded for successes and mildly chastised for failures. People find the ongoing personal contacts and longstanding friendships rewarding. Many members are motivated to lose weight because of their empathy for one another.

The TOPS approach has been repeated by many organizations both voluntary and commercial all over North America. Their success at helping people overcome weight problems varies from community to community.

It is my opinion that the organizations with the best success rate at helping people lose weight are the volunteer groups that emphasize maturity and independence as qualities to strive for during and after weight loss.

A relatively new organization patterned after Alcoholics Anonymous is aimed altogether at using your head. AA uses personal success testimonials for inspiring other people, and Overeaters Anonymous follows the same approach. I have heard many reports of praise and a few specific criticisms about this strictly noncommercial organization.

Personal testimonials by people with similar eating problems help you get rid of your feelings of being the only one with a particular eating problem.

Solutions to specific eating and food problems are freely shared in testimonials and widen your own possibilities for solution.

There is no weighing-in at the meetings and no chastising of any kind, so there's no element of guilt or embarrassment before other people. Guilt feelings rob you of maturity and make you feel dependent and detract from your self-esteem.

Problems and effective ways to handle them are shared on a first-name-only basis. Everyone is free to speak at will.

The meetings are free of charge except for a voluntary donation to cover the cost of phone calls and post cards to announce future meetings.

When I attended Overeaters Anonymous meetings to observe, I saw slim people get up to say they'd been helped by OA and wanted to continue coming to meetings to prevent backsliding.

I have heard two specific criticisms of OA. One is that people get up and give self-styled medical advice that listeners don't know whether to believe or not. The other criticism is that sometimes the meetings have too many people from one ethnic group. Personal testimonies describing eating binges of ethnic foods are hard to understand if you are not familiar with those foods. But I also heard people asking what was in such and such food. How much fat? How many calories? How do you fix it? What does it taste like? So in the end, everyone understood the composition of the high-calorie ethnic dishes. I heard several people comment on how much they had learned.

The all-day marathon in a large public hall is an OA innovation. I attended a twelve-hour weekend marathon and heard testimonials from people who work on weekdays—people who had come to recognize their problem as exhaustion-adrenalin-hypoglycemia eating. These people varied from moonlighters to mothers of small children who worked long hours, prodded by *nerve,* and who ate one long meal from dinner to bedtime.

Here are two unusual testimonials.

A salesman told how he'd quit smoking when his father died of lung cancer. He said he switched to filled cookies, which he kept on the seat of his car and nibbled as he drove between his accounts. Two years and twenty pounds later, he said, an insurance physical discovered sugar in his urine. "My doctor put me on a diet, but I forgot to mention the cookies. They were such a habit, I took them for granted. When I didn't lose weight, the doctor suggested I keep a food diary. Then I *discovered* the cookies. I tried to quit, cold turkey, but after the first day, I knew I wouldn't make it. I had gone to an OA meeting with a friend where I got the idea of bringing a bag of raw carrots from home to nibble on. After about a month, I was much better. My doctor explained how the sugar I was eating drove my blood sugar up, which caused my pancreas to make more insulin, which drove my blood sugar way down and made me feel hungry again right away."

A part-time actress, who said she was a crowd-scene ham, explained that in between jobs she sat home, ate, and nervously waited for casting departments to call. "One year when work was slow," she said, "I gained ten pounds in three months of waiting for the phone to ring. I was well on the way to being a *foodaholic.* I knew all the signs because I had been overweight as a teenager. I knew how to diet from my teen experience, and began to plan all my meals ahead, write out menus, and vow to stick to them. In order to keep myself out of the kitchen between meals and get more exercise, I decided to paint and redecorate my apartment."

Both said that hearing other peoples' problems helped them build up their will power to fight off backsliding.

Any religious or community organization with a large public room could provide meeting space for this type of *nonprofit self-help through group inspiration.*

YOUR GOAL: A SOUND MIND IN A SOUND BODY

Ideally, your body will decide when to eat and when to stop. But if you are like many people, living in an abundant society that presses food on you constantly, your head must intervene.

When the eating urge overpowers all efforts at self-assessment and self-control, powerful psychological factors may underlie your troubles. This does not make weight loss impossible. Basic retraining of many years of bad habits is still the practical objective whether or not you need professional treatment.

When hunger, satisfaction, food, and eating are closely woven into severe emotional disturbances, I advise psychiatric or psychological help.

Our society has a brutally negative and hostile attitude toward overweight people. Overly sensitive and vulnerable personalities are very likely to suffer emotionally from this attitude.

But you can lose weight—on your own, or with the help of friends or professionals. And the goal is to lose it, maintain a new desirable weight for life, and not go overboard by getting too thin.

The next thing you have to do is make a plan for personal food control, based completely on your own life style, genetics, and your reasons for wanting to lose weight.

Be practical and realistic. Fad diets are not the answer. Use your head.

ARE THERE MAGIC FORMULAS FOR WEIGHT LOSS?

Diets and Dieting

STOP DIETING—START EATING TO LIVE

Are you a guinea pig? Chances are you've never thought about reducing diets as an experiment on you. But this is the way it turns out if you are one of millions of people who try a fad diet or a crash diet.

A *fad* diet is one that tells you what to eat.

A *crash* diet is one that is low in calories to bring about fast weight loss.

A diet can be both *fad* and *crash*. *Fad* stands for the food part and *crash* for the time you stay on the diet.

Over 100 million human guinea pigs have tried fad or crash diets and at the same time have helped build up scientific data on what the diets do to the human body.

What do the data show?

First, you have to divide the data into two parts: How effective is the diet for weight loss? And how good or bad is the diet for health?

Anyone can lose weight on any fad diet, so weight loss alone isn't the issue. The issue is that unless they need to lose only a few pounds, people rarely achieve their desired weight goal. After stopping the fad diet, most people gain the weight back and often go on to gain more.

Do you have a closetful of clothes of various sizes that you bought when your weight was going up and down? You have plenty of company, because fad diets bring about the "yo-yo syndrome." This term was devised by a man who claimed to have gained and lost 1,000 pounds.

What Is the Matter with Reducing Diets?

Reducing diets fail to inform you that the only road to sustained weight loss is *your total, conscious control of everything connected with eating.*

Reducing diets fail to *instruct* your appetite-fullness habits.

They fail to teach you how to eat to live instead of living to eat.

They have poor results for ideal weight loss and even poorer results for maintenance of ideal weight.

They fail to tell you how and why they work. They leave you confused, thinking something *in you* caused failure.

Modern high-density foods are so plentiful, tempting, and tasty, you have to learn a whole new way to cope with eating. Dieting is not enough.

Weight loss is the primary purpose of a reducing diet, but for many years it was essential for a diet to be pleasant and easy to take. On the surface, there is nothing wrong with this. Beneath the surface, however, many fad diets prove to have predictable health hazards. The hazards are serious for people with genetic susceptibilities. But *susceptibilities without known hereditary causes also show up.*

All of us cannot eat the same way and be healthy. For good health, your food choices need to be compatible with your body chemistry. For you to lose weight, your food-intake calories need to be fewer than the calories you burn for energy.

It is completely up to you to decide whether you want to be thin and healthy. But this goal requires you *to make up your mind to like and to eat the foods best suited for your chemistry.*

Your body chemistry is a mixture of genetic traits, individual tendencies, and special needs, such as growth, and stages of life such as pregnancy and menopause (male and female). Your body chemistry is also affected by your sex, age, and any illness you may have. Your health may be better in the long run if you adopt a whole new approach to eating instead of going on an occasional fad diet or fast.

A new lifetime way of eating means you have to know *why* you eat the foods you eat. The better you know *why,* the more likely you are to keep your weight where you want it. It's the same idea as knowing why you want to lose weight. Increased knowledge will pay off in increased will power— if you find out how each type of food works in your body and why it works that way. It will help you avoid being a guinea pig the next time an old diet comes out under a new name.

The only way to solve your weight problem is to be in continuous conscious control of everything connected with food and eating.

Thousands of weight-loss diets have appeared in magazines, books, and newspapers. Does it surprise you to find out that they can be grouped into as few as eight categories? Well, they can be: high-protein diets, high-fat diets, low-carbohydrate diets, one-food diets, fasting diets, low-calorie balanced diets, gimmick diets, and high-fiber diets.

HIGH-PROTEIN DIETS

The first fad diet came out in England in 1864. William Banting, who weighed over 200 pounds, was advised by his physician Sir William Harvey to eat only meat. Sir William got the idea from the renowned French physiologist Claude Bernard, who taught Sir William that removing all sugar from the diet helped diabetes. Sir William decided that the ultimate in a no-sugar diet was an all-meat diet. The patient, William Banting, was delighted by his loss of thirty-five pounds in thirty-eight days and wrote a little pamphlet called *Letter on Corpulence,* published in London in 1864.

Since that time, there has been a long parade of high-protein diets. Why?

High-protein diets owe much of their popularity to quick weight loss. These diets burn protein in the body and leave a large amount of acid. The body washes out the acid with water. Water loss accounts for rapid weight reduction on the scale. Scale weight has a powerful effect on morale.

By the end of the first week, water loss decreases. What happens next? By then, many dieters have lost their appetite. Those who persist on the diet have no trouble eating less than 1,200 to 1,500 calories a day. If they can continue on the diet, they will eventually lose fat, though fat loss takes place much more slowly than water loss.

Have you ever tried a high-protein diet? You will remember that by the end of the first week, you felt rotten. You probably had a giddy feeling, frequently became sick to your stomach, and were weak and tired.

If you did what most people do at that point, you ate some carbohydrate food. Only fifty grams of carbohydrate stops the water loss of a high-protein diet and makes you feel better. Fifty grams of carbohydrate is contained, for example, in two large apples or one small serving of layer cake.

After you stop a high-protein diet, you feel better because there is less acid in your body. The acid condition is called *ketosis.*

If you believe that ketosis has its good points because it wrecks your appetite, you are right. But there are certain people whose health is harmed by ketosis, and they should never undertake a diet that causes ketosis without being aware of the hazards.

Ketosis can be associated with hypoglycemia from dieting.* Hypoglycemia stimulates adrenalin formation in the body. Adrenalin brings on blood-pressure elevation. And even though the elevation is temporary, it is unhealthful for people with hypertension and heart disease.

When a woman is pregnant, adrenalin formation can harm the unborn child because adrenalin decreases the blood flow to the uterus and diverts it to the mother's skeletal muscles. If a pregnant woman has ketosis, her

---

*This ketosis is not the same as the keto-acidosis in severe diabetes.

unborn child is robbed of blood supply. This decreased blood flow is only temporary, but if it occurs during the time that an important part of the baby's body is being formed, birth defects can result. Unborn children are especially susceptible to harm from any diet that causes ketosis. This susceptibility has nothing to do with heredity; it has everything to do with the unique chemistry of fetal development.

People with diabetes are especially susceptible to ketosis and should not try diets that cause it.

Ketosis from an acid diet tends to pull calcium out of the bones. People who are susceptible to kidney stones should stay away from any diet that pulls calcium out of the bones.

A painful condition called *osteoporosis* is the result of decreased calcium in the bones, especially the spinal bones, or vertebrae. Bones become soft and break easily from minor accidents. Osteoporosis is the main cause of broken bones from minor accidents among older people. Osteoporosis is becoming more common in a special susceptibility group, *postmenopausal women.* It also occurs in older men, but is less common than in women.

I suspect that ketosis-causing fad diets are responsible for some of the increase of this crippling disease. In the past two decades, the popular ways to lose weight have featured the ketosis-causing diets with little or no exercise.

Exercise helps a great deal to keep the calcium in the bones where it belongs. Ketosis and no exercise are an unhealthful combination for bones, especially women's bones.

If you have a family history of osteoporosis or kidney stones or any calcium disease, your best bet is to leave ketosis-causing diets to guinea pigs.

Ketosis causes sticky blood, just as elevated blood triglycerides do.

Birth control pills and estrogen pills also cause sticky blood. A ketogenic diet combined with one of these medications gives you extra chances for suffering a blood clot in the lungs or a stroke.

If you have no special susceptibilities to ketogenic diseases, you still should know several facts before deciding to follow a high-protein diet.

Most high-protein diets are also high-fat diets. High-fat diets overload the metabolism even though you eat fewer calories than you burn. Even with meats carefully trimmed, poultry skin removed, no fats added, and no food fried, self-selected high-protein diets still turn out to be high in fat.

A Harvard University research team made a careful study of an enormously popular high-protein diet.* The diet suggests that you eat all you want of meat, poultry, fish, seafood, eggs, low-fat cheese, and dairy products. Look at the average daily food selection made by Harvard students who were the volunteers studied by the Harvard researchers:

*The Stillman Diet, Number 1, see page 90.

6 ounces of beef or lamb
3 ounces of fish or seafood
3 ounces of chicken or turkey
1½ cups of cottage cheese or other allowed cheese
2½ eggs

If you calculate the amounts of protein, fat, and carbohydrate in these foods, as the Harvard study did, you will find that the total foods constitute a high-fat diet. The following table shows the amounts of fat, protein, and carbohydrate that the Harvard students ate.

The amounts of fat, protein, and carbohydrate are shown in three different ways—grams, ounces, and in calories:

TOTAL FAT	TOTAL PROTEIN
73 grams plus 7 grams of cholesterol	160 grams
2½ ounces plus ¼ ounce of cholesterol	5 ounces
720 calories	640 calories

TOTAL CHOLESTEROL	TOTAL CARBOHYDRATE
(Separated from total fat to emphasize how high it is.)	(The only carbohydrate is milk sugar.)
7 grams	12 grams
¼ ounce	½ ounce
63 calories	48 calories

True, 1,419 total calories is reasonable for an average reducing diet. But this is deceptive because over 50 percent of the calories is fat.

Fat-susceptible people make too much endogenous cholesterol out of the fat they eat. This is especially true when they eat saturated fat. The American Heart Association tells fat-susceptible people to eat less than 300 milligrams a day of exogenous cholesterol. These people make endogenous cholesterol so readily, especially from saturated fat, that their total cholesterol can quickly get too high. Most of the fat in the self-selected high-fat diet is saturated fat.

Daily intake of 7,000 milligrams, or 7 grams, of exogenous food cholesterol is dangerously high for fat-susceptible people.

All of the Harvard volunteers who ate this diet ended up with elevated blood cholesterol. None of the volunteers was known to be especially fat-sensitive, and being college students, their genetic weaknesses were minimized by youth. You can see that you have to look into more than just calories when it comes to healthful eating for weight loss. What are *your* chances of having a genetic fat susceptibility?

Gout—another inherited susceptibility—surfaces from high-protein diets. Many people in North America have a genetic tendency for gout without being aware of it. This is called *silent gout.*

One day Vera C., one of my patients, was dusting the tops of her drapery valences. She slipped and fell off a twelve-inch stepladder and accidently kicked the ladder with one foot on her way down. The foot that hit the ladder began to swell right away. By the next day it was huge, angry, red, and painful. Vera was sure she had a broken bone in her foot but the X-ray showed no fracture. Instead, the X-ray showed many little round punched-out bubbles. This is the X-ray look of gout.

Vera had been overweight most of her life; most of her family was overweight. Fortunately, Vera was not interested in fad diets or her gout would have surfaced earlier. The key thing is that Vera had no knowledge of a family history of gout. It is likely that gout would be found in family members, were they to look for it.

Cholesterol diseases, diabetes, and gout are becoming so common in the United States and Canada that diets that cause them to surface should throw up a stop sign in your mind.

TABLE 1. HIGH-PROTEIN DIETS*

Title	Chief Characteristics
Banting-Harvey	England, 1864; meat, mutton, bacon; as little as possible of bread, milk, butter, beer, sugar.
Earl of Salisbury	England, 1890's; ground beef (given the name Salisbury steak).
Pennington, also known as Du Pont	A fat-meat diet; each meal consisted of 2 to 3 ounces of fat and 6 to 9 ounces of meat.
Stillman Diet, Number 1	All you want of lean meats and poultry, lean fish and seafood, eggs, and low-fat cheeses; required to drink 8 glasses of water, take daily vitamin supplements; no refined flour, sugar, alcohol, or whole-milk products.
Stillman Diet, Number 2	1,125 calories; 25 grams of carbohydrate, 25 grams of fat, 200 grams of protein. The author states that people told him they had to have some carbohydrate, at least a tossed salad. A few exercises are added; 10 glasses of sugar-free water (coffee, tea, or soda).
Fat Free Forever Elting and Isenberg	Essentially the same as the Stillman Diet, Number 2.
Born to be Fat Friedman	Essentially the same as the Stillman Diet, Number 2, with the added idea that some people have no recourse, as they were born to be fat.

*Here, and for the sections that follow, see Bibliography for complete details on sources.

Diet Is Not Enough Perlstein	Remove all the visible fat; then eat all the meat and fish you can eat three times a day; plus exercise; shun pills and keep calm.
Weighing Game Riccio and Riccio	High-protein, low-fat, minimum processed food, exercise, six small meals a day and no calorie counting. Recommended snacks: Soybeans, raisins, nuts. While good for you, these are high-calorie.
Natural Food, High Protein Recipes Hayden	High-protein recipes; ingredients consist of natural foods and soy flour, wheat germ, yogurt, cottage cheese.
Hauser	A pioneer of low-fat milk and dairy products, low-fat yogurt—1 quart a day to decrease appetite—plus eggs, lean meat, and cottage cheese; high in raw vegetables; low fruit because of fruit sugar; no refined sugar or flour.
Lazy Lady Petrie	High-protein; low in refined flour, sugar, potatoes; instead of counting calories, count points assigned by Petrie. Claims protein is "miracle weight reducer." Later modification: Start with fruit and work up to high-protein.
Remarkable Ratio de Ville	The higher the protein content to the given number of calories the better; gives a list of ratios for common foods: Eat low-numbered foods; a bit of skim milk or a tablespoon of polyunsaturated fats daily; take vitamins; drink lots of water.
Low Carbohydrate Fredericks	High-protein, moderately high fat, one-fifth of which should be polyunsaturated oils; no calorie counting; six meals a day. This diet belongs on both high-protein and high-fat lists. Fredericks has more recently advocated the high-fiber approach.
Nova Scotia	Supposed to have originated at Camp Hill, Nova Scotia. All fish and seafood; implies no frying, therefore no fat, few calories. Easy, as few foods are involved.
Yogurt Diet	Plain yogurt, slice in your own fruit; commercial fruited yogurt has added refined sugar, so calorie count is double that of plain yogurt; contains saturated fats if made from whole milk; however, calorie count is easy because few foods are involved.
No Will Power (Ladies' Home Journal), Wisconsin (after a study done at the Univ. of Wisconsin) and Petrie also has one of these.	These are basically nibbling diets; some advocate starting with a day or two of fasting; very light breakfast as this is often a low hunger time of day. Calorie count is fairly simple; moderate number of foods; salad advocated in addition to high protein.
Nine Day Wonder Diet, New Nine Day Wonder Diet	Claim you will lose nine pounds in nine days; basically high-protein, low-calorie; the 1940 version has about 800 calories; the 1974 version has 1,200 calories and some thought is given to saturated fat.
Olympic Diet	Developed for the Women's Alpine Team. Very similar to the Nine-Day and New Nine-Day. Very light breakfast, high-protein lunch and dinner with some low-calorie carbohydrate and a little fat (olives); diet tells you what to eat at each meal on each day of the week.

HIGH-FAT DIETS

From looking at the foods, it's hard to tell the difference between high-protein diets and high-fat diets. The protein foods that come from animals are almost half fat. A small serving of animal protein food—steak, ribs, cold cuts, or frankfurters—contains seven grams of protein and five grams of fat. It is faulty thinking to ignore this fact when you are dealing with weight loss.

Translated into calories, a one-ounce portion of animal protein, three inches long, two inches wide, and one-eighth inch thick, has twenty-eight calories of protein and forty-five calories of fat. Chicken and other fowl have less fat, but you have to remove the skin. Bacon is considered a *fat* food.

Chocolate, cream cheese, mayonnaise, nuts, olives, and avocado are also considered to be fat foods. These, with animal proteins, are included in high-fat diets.

High-fat diets, like high-protein diets, leave a large amount of acid when they burn in the body. Like high-protein diets, high-fat diets cause ketosis and loss of appetite, fatigue, and hypoglycemia.

Overloaded fat metabolism, elevated blood cholesterol, and triglycerides always come with a high-fat diet.

Even if polyunsaturated vegetable fat is substituted when possible, elevations of cholesterol and triglyceride show that metabolism is overloaded. People with inherited susceptibilities show signs of overloading sooner, and their blood cholesterol and triglycerides go up higher.

High-fat diets are dangerous for fat-susceptible people. If you have any of the susceptibilities to trouble from ketosis or overloaded fat metabolism, beware of high-fat diets.

The following are high-fat diets popular in past decades. Despite all the health drawbacks for many North Americans, other high-fat diets may appear.

TABLE 2. HIGH-FAT DIETS

Title	Chief Characteristics
Pennington: The Du Pont Diet Thorpe	Fat-meat diet; actually high-fat, high-protein. Theory is that overweight people "turn too much carbohydrate into fat." Recommendation is three parts of meat to one of fat: meat, 3 grams, to fat, 1 gram. A later version of the diet added suet—high in saturated fat.
Eat, Drink and Get Thin Reinsh	This diet calls for eating all the fat meat you want; claims it is an ideal fuel for the body's furnace and that it burns off excess starch and avoids water logging. Also claims that iodized salt has suppressed thyroid

function even though it reduced the incidence of goiter. I know of no medical evidence to show that the usual amounts of iodized salt can depress the function of the normal thyroid gland. Forbidden foods are potatoes, cereals, flour products, ice cream, candy, soft drinks, highly salted foods; alcohol is permitted in moderation, sweet cordials, however, are taboo. Fluids are restricted to 1½ quarts a day. Exercise is recommended. Permits all meat, no matter how fatty, all fish, all seafood, butter, lard, margarine, oils, cream, salad dressing, and all vegetables except potatoes. Note that if enough of the permitted fruits and vegetables are taken with this diet, the ketosis of a high-fat diet might be prevented; however, if the total calories of food eaten are low enough for fat loss, ketosis could still result. However, the diet retains the inherent problems of increasing the amount of total fat in the circulation.

Calories Don't Count
Taller

High-fat diet that coincided with the general knowledge explosion of unsaturation versus saturation of fats. Same initial salt and water loss as any high-fat diet; same ketosis, leading to decreased appetite. Biochemical theory of "fat balance" never agreed to by anyone except Taller. This author and his theories lost popularity when he was charged in Federal Court in connection with a tie-in with a company selling the same brand of safflower-oil capsules recommended in the book.

Eat and Become Slim—a Beauty Diet With Vegetable Oil
Arai

Chinese cooking forms the basis of much of this diet: Cook with vegetable oil from corn, cottonseed, rice, safflower, sesame, and sunflower. Animal fat—lard, butter—are taboo. Basis is that carbohydrates stimulate appetite by remaining in the stomach only three hours while fat remains for five hours, thus decreasing hunger. (Note: Experiments show stomach-emptying time is not important as a cause of hunger.)

The Boston Police Diet
Berman

High in saturated fat, free of all sugar; milk taboo because it contains milk sugar; deep frying is taboo. Suggests thyroid pills to be prescribed by your doctor. This diet was "officially renounced by the Boston Police Department." (*Consumer's Guide,* "Rating the Diets," April 1975.)

Diet Revolution
Atkins

Eat all you want of bacon and eggs, seafood and chicken salad with mayonnaise, seafood with lemon-butter sauce, cheese omelet with bacon, and eggs Benedict with Hollandaise sauce, and so on. Snacks consist of cheese, cold cuts, cold shrimp, cottage cheese, creamy ricotta cheese enhanced with artificial sweeteners and flavorings as desired. No fruits, vegetables, sugars, starches, breads, sweet pickles, chewing gum, ice cream, catsup, and so on. The advised objective is ketosis; after a week or so of ketosis and desired weight loss, diet adds a few carbohydrate and protein foods, mostly low-calorie, but also a few "prizes" such as cheese cake and a little alcohol. The diet advises its followers to test urine with ketone-testing chemical: Gross sales of Ketostix went up $3 million in 1973. Author criticized in medical, public health, and nutrition publications.

LOW-CARBOHYDRATE DIETS

Low-carbohydrate diets are high-fat diets in disguise. They appeared on the scene in the 1960s and started in the United Kingdom where more refined sugar is eaten per capita than anywhere else in the world. North America runs a close second.

The low-carbohydrate approach to weight loss gives the impression that all carbohydrate foods are heavy in calories and bad for you. This is incorrect. Fruits, vegetables, grains, and roots are carbohydrates. These are high-volume, low-density foods so long as they are not prepared or processed with fats or sugars (see page 205).

The biggest calorie excesses in advanced civilizations come from sugar and fat. Here is where the trouble lies. These foods are so palatable, they are habit-forming. They are so widely available, so easy to grab, they spell trouble.

The purpose of the low-carbohydrate diet was to call these things to your attention. The low-carbohydrate diets did add to the number of people who question how much sugar they should eat.

But on the whole, low-carbohydrate diets fail to make any inroads in the overweight problem. They end up being high-fat diets. They are unhealthful for people who are ketosis-sensitive (see page 87) and for everybody whose brain is affected by symptoms of hypoglycemia.

The hypoglycemic effect comes on when you have ketosis. You feel faint, headachy, have a stomachache or a cheap high. Your brain doesn't feel hungry when you have hypoglycemia caused by ketosis because you are sick to your stomach. You can faint, you can easily get into an auto accident or a work or home accident when your brain is not getting enough glucose.

Hypoglycemia makes the brain unusually sensitive to alcohol and can cause drunkenness in people who consume as little as one and a half ounces of alcohol. This is a big hazard.

People with hypertension should beware of the hypoglycemia-adrenalin effect. Hypoglycemia, brought on by ketosis, causes adrenalin production. Those who make a lot of adrenalin are very susceptible to this effect. But hypoglycemia causes adrenalin production even if you are calm and free from tension and worries. This adrenalin is used to get glucose to your brain fast. At the same time, adrenalin raises blood pressure and constricts coronary and brain arteries.

People with cholesterol plaques in their important arteries should beware of the hypoglycemia-adrenalin effect. Adrenalin can fully shut off coronary blood flow.

For people with diabetes, ketosis can quickly be complicated by diabetic coma.

Because they are high-fat diets, low-carbohydrate diets are not healthful for people with inherited weakness from overloaded fat metabolism. They can result in big increases of blood cholesterol.

Besides causing ketosis and fat overloading, low-carbohydrate diets fail overweight people in other ways:

The diets have gimmicks that confuse the already complex subject of what to eat in order to lose weight. Gimmicks give the impression that some magic ingredient will whisk unwanted weight away.

Nothing will whisk unwanted fat away. The only thing that will get rid of unwanted fat is steady, day-to-day expending of more energy than you take in as food.

The low-carbohydrate diets use contrived formulas, called "carbo-cals." or "carbo-calories" to guide daily food choices. Faddish calculations put the emphasis on tricks instead of on the central fact.

The central fact is that one average serving of dessert—pie, cake, or ice cream—is so loaded with calories that right there is *one-third* of your daily food intake. These desserts have between 400 and 500 calories. If that dessert will keep you full and satisfied for twenty-four hours, you probably don't have a weight problem. Most of us need to eat a much greater volume of food to feel satisfied.

To those who really want to lose weight, it is much more realistic to say: Eat only fruit, fresh or prepared without added sugar, for dessert. Or, to put it right on the line: If you have a sweet tooth, if rich desserts are among your favorite foods, you have to give them up, at least for the time being. *You have to give up foods that urge you to eat more* (see p. 8).

When can you try them again? When you get to the point where you can skimp to save calories for a special treat. When you can eat one—and only one—tablespoonful of a food that urges you to eat more, just to get the taste sensation. When you get to your ideal weight and want to splurge once or twice a year on very special holidays.

The chief examples of low-carbohydrate diets are presented so you will be able to recognize this high-fat diet in disguise when you see it.

TABLE 3. LOW-CARBOHYDRATE DIETS

Title	Chief Characteristics
Low Carbohydrate Diet Yudkin	Count carbohydrates instead of calories; gives a table called carbohydrate units or or CU (one CU is actually about 5 grams of carbohydrate); you are limited to

eating 10 CU a day, which is 50 grams of carbohydrates. The only dietary concern is sugar; recommends far less than current high-sugar consumption in Western diets, little or no bread, one small potato or none; fruits and vegetables not condemned, but sugar is not to be added in any form. Intended by Dr. Yudkin to be a "sound, nutritious eating program." In practice, it often became a high-fat, high-protein diet, because food selection recommendations stress fat meat and other fatty foods.

Drinking Man's Diet
"Jameson and Williams," pseudonyms of freelance writer, Robert Wernick

An alcoholic version of the low-carbohydrate diet with the cautioning advice to eat at least 30 grams of carbohydrate a day. Advice against gorging: "If you gorge yourself with food, even if it is low in carbohydrates, you will get fat." According to review in *Time* magazine: "The book's contents are a cocktail of wishful thinking, jigger of nonsense, and a dash of sound advice."

Carbo-Cal
Petrie

Takes the carbohydrate content of food and gives it to you in terms of calories, based on carbohydrate's supplying 4 calories per gram; a gimmick.

Thinking Man's Diet
McMahon

Follows *Carbo-Cal;* allows 60 grams of carbohydrate; a gimmick.

Carbo-Calorie
Mart

Gives a formula for combining a unit of heat and a unit of weight, explains that this is an artificial measurement: $20a + b \div 24 = X$, a is carbohydrate count in grams, b the calorie count, and x the Carbo-Calorie count. Using this scheme, 100 Carbo-Cals provide 60 grams of carbohydrate and 1,200 calories. Recommended daily diet of 58 Carbo-Cals provides 30 grams of carbohydrate and 800 calories; also advises preparation of balanced menus, added vitamins; before dieting, consult your doctor, and take the book along wherever you go.

Low-Carbo Diet
Tarr Natural Foods

Calls attention to many natural foods; is against processed foods; unique recipes; limits carbohydrates to 58 grams daily; wrong information: "Without carbohydrates you cannot gain weight."

Fat Destroyer Foods
Petrie and Stone

Gives diets of varying carbohydrate content all the way up to no carbohydrate, nearly 100 percent fat and protein.

MONOTONOUS ONE-FOOD DIETS

The purpose of monotonous one-food diets is to remove *dieting* completely from ordinary living.

You don't have to think about what you eat.

You don't have to think about what *not* to eat.

Food is a nutritional experiment instead of *just eating*.

The first monotonous one-food diet for weight reduction was the forerunner of the formula diet. This came out in the 1860s when a doctor prescribed a diet limited to four glasses of creamy milk a day.

In the 1940s, a medically supervised formula diet was worked out at a New York hospital. The formula was a mixture of canned evaporated milk, glucose (body sugar), and corn oil. It was flavored with a small amount of vanilla and provided 750 calories a day. The whole mixture was diluted with water and usually served over ice. The water and ice were to supply the kidneys with enough water to do their work efficiently. The cracked ice also helped create the fantasy of drinking an ice-cream soda instead of a medical reducing formula.

The 750 calories were divided into ten to twelve daily *doses* because small, frequent feedings best satisfy the appetite.

Soon the formula was commercialized. You can still buy versions of it in supermarkets and drugstores.

Milk products are high-protein foods that do not cause ketosis because there is enough milk sugar (lactose) to counterbalance the protein-acid ash. The added glucose in the formula ensures against ketosis.

A short-term formula diet for up to two weeks or so is still a good way to lose a few pounds. But you haven't learned anything from it, and it keeps feeding your sweet tooth.

Substituting one can of formula (250 calories) or one solid diet bar (250 calories) for one meal also feeds your sweet tooth, a practice to be avoided.

Formula feedings are low in iron; people with low-iron weakness, beware.

People with milk intolerance from lactase deficiency or allergy beware.

The rice diet, an extreme one-food diet for greatly overweight people, was developed by a prestigious medical specialist in hypertension, heart disease, and kidney disease. The rice diet proved that most overweight people do not need added salt in their diet. It has also shown that the more overweight people are, the less protein they need.

The rice diet also proved that anyone can lose weight all the way down to ideal weight for height.

The rice diet consists of 400 to 800 calories a day of boiled rice, without added salt, and some fresh fruit in season. The small amount of fresh fruit means the diet is not quite one food. But it is still monotonous to people who are overweight from eating high-density foods that tempt them to eat more and more. Drinking lots of water is encouraged. Daily multivitamins are recommended. (Vitamins are recommended with any extreme diet.)

Reasonably active* overweight people will lose weight at about 1200 to

---

*Overweight persons at complete bed rest will not lose weight unless their calories are cut to 800 or less.

1500 calories per day. Lowering food calories to one-half or one-third of these amounts will cause ketosis on high-protein, high-fat, and low-carbohydrate diets. Ketosis does not occur on the rice diet because it is counteracted by rice and fruit, which are nearly all carbohydrate.

The rice diet has been immensely successful in the hands of medical specialists at Duke University in Durham, North Carolina. Patients are encouraged to take long, daily walks. These men and women are not hospitalized; they live independently and have only to report to the outpatient clinic for daily blood-pressure checks and motivational talks.

Under medical supervision, the rice diet is simple and safe. The only medical drawback is for people who must have protein in their diets. However, after two or three months a very small amount of lean meat or poultry is added. Often a small amount of vegetable is added after one month.

Grossly overweight people, nearly 400 pounds or more, have stayed on the rice diet for as long as twelve and one-half months, losing as much as 275 pounds. The average weight loss, overall, is about 140 pounds. Many people have achieved their ideal weights.

There is, however, an economic drawback. It's costly to leave home and go to live for several months in Durham, North Carolina. There are the medical fees, too. But this method of weight loss is cheaper and far safer than intestinal bypass surgery (see pages 129–130). Neither method can promise lifetime weight loss. Some people go home from the rice diet at their ideal weight and gain weight at home. The rice diet does have more success than surgery at bringing people to ideal weight.

Both methods are, however, removed from everyday living. Both put attention on weight loss instead of on what's going to happen in real life when you're again faced with the foods that urge you to eat more.

There *is* room for extreme methods for extremely overweight people. Before the rice diet was used for weight loss, it was used successfully with seriously ill people with hypertension and heart disease, who often are overweight. The success of the diet in the disease treatment was always accompanied by weight loss. This is how the rice diet came to be used for treating extreme overweight.

There are any number of other monotonous one-food diets. They are mostly insignificant, and some are silly and were meant to capture an audience of people who were looking for magic. There is no magic or mystery about weight problems. There is no food that has special fat-burning properties. Forget it.

All a diet does is reinforce strict calorie counting. It does this by getting you to make a contract with yourself to pass up all other foods except those the diet calls for.

If you want some one- or two-week quickie diets to lose a few pounds that you picked up on a cruise or at a round of parties, try a monotonous one-food diet. Be sure it won't do you harm from the genetic food-chemistry or bad-habit angle.

Here is a very simple one-food monotonous diet: Drink six 8-ounce glasses of nonfat milk a day. You can flavor the milk with coffee, tea, vanilla, nutmeg, lemon, or orange. These must be flavorings, not juices or syrups, all of which contain sugar calories.

Each eight-ounce glass contains 80 calories. Milk lacks iron and vitamin C, but a week or two will not be harmful unless you are pregnant or nursing.

People with lactase deficiency, who can't digest milk, can substitute yogurt.

Here is an idea of what most of the monotonous one-food diets are like:

TABLE 4. MONOTONOUS ONE-FOOD DIETS

Title	Chief Characteristics
Liquid-formula Diets—succeeded by Diet Bars (a solid version of the formula)	Formula diets were originally mixed by hospital nutrition departments. The simple sugar glucose (syn. dextrose), the sugar in human blood, was used instead of sucrose because it was considered to be more natural. Later, the pharmaceutical companies made these formulas in flavored varieties available on the commercial market. From these, followed a solid pastry or cookie version. Each portion has a calorie count—the idea being that if you eat, say, four of these a day, one every three hours until bedtime, you will have ingested 250 calories of food energy four times, or 1,000 calories, and would not allow yourself "the temptation of real food." Some people have been confused by these, thinking that some magic or special ingredient in the formula food would allow them to lose weight while they continued to eat their usual food. Formulas which are based on whole milk are high in exogenous cholesterol and saturated fat. Fat- and cholesterol-susceptible people take note. People with lactose intolerance often suffer diarrhea and cramps from these formulas. However, for many overweight people, the formula diet is harmless for a week or two.
Ice Cream and Ice-Cream Soda Diets	Scoop of vanilla ice cream with or without soda water, three to four times a day: 500 to 750 calories; may decrease ice-cream craving or may make it worse.
Hard-Boiled Egg Diet	One to 10 eggs a day, one every hour; high in exogenous cholesterol, constipating, ketosis-predisposing diet. Use of egg substitute eliminates cholesterol, but it can't be hard-boiled. The theory that protein increased heat loss became obsolete after these diets were popular.
Grapefruit Diet, Apple Diet, Tomato-Juice Diet	People who supported the grapefruit diet claimed that grapefruit had some special fat-burning property. This is not true. The fact is, though, that a grapefruit every hour for twelve hours will keep you busy and satisfied

for only 500 to 600 calories of food energy a day.
Tomato juice has about the same calories as grapefruit.
Apples have about one-third more calories. All these
are antiketogenic.

FASTING

You need to think about fasting in two ways. There is fasting you can do
on your own, and there is medically supervised fasting. A fast of more than
one day can be unhealthful for susceptible people. And there are many
people in North America whose health could be affected adversely by
fasting.

Fasting causes ketosis. All people easily subject to ketosis should get
medical advice before fasting. Pregnant women should never fast without
medical advice. People with cholesterol plaques in their coronary arteries
should not fast. Remember how ketosis brings about the hypoglycemia-
adrenalin response.

Even though the human body was programmed for alternate feast and
famine, we have progressed beyond the point where human life is expend-
able. Fasting of more than a day is a very individual thing in our society.

The protein-sparing modified fast (PSMF), now becoming a fad, is really
a version of the monotony diet. In some, casein (milk protein) and glucose
are mixed and given in daily doses of 250 to 300 calories. In others, purified
amino-acid mixtures are used instead of milk protein.

The PSMF can cause ketosis in susceptible people and can worsen kidney
trouble. The PSMF was meant to be used by physicians for treating extremely overweight people in a hospital. Its use is controversial among
doctors. It will not help you learn better food and eating habits for a
lifetime.

If you don't have a health or safety reason for not fasting, you can still
run into problems. The problems are in your hunger and your eating habits.

I often come across people who try to lose weight by fasting for one day
a week. The next day they usually make up for it. They say they can't stop
eating. These are usually people whose bodies are very resistant to ketosis;
ketosis itself decreases appetite.

But there's no advantage to fasting for a day and then making up for it
the next. And what's more important, over the long haul, you haven't
learned anything about better ways to choose and eat foods.

What is medically supervised fasting? This is fasting that can last for
several days up to seven or eight weeks.* *Total fasting,* when only water

*The world's record, a very unusual occurrence, is nearly four months.

is taken, means that all the energy the body needs for its daily functioning comes from within the body. The 1,200 to 1,500 calories that the fasting person needs for a moderately sedentary day comes from the fat stores and later on from the fat-cell walls.

Individual susceptibilities, such as gout and anemia, can surface during a long fast. One of the responsibilities of the doctor attending a fasting patient is to be on the lookout for these diseases as well as for complications from ketosis.

An early goal in a supervised fast is to get patients started on daily walks in order to increase their calorie output. Often, patients seriously ill with diabetes, hypertension, and heart disease feel better and start walking as soon as they've dropped ten pounds.

Long-term medically supervised fasts are for people who have health complications and thirty to fifty pounds or more to lose. People of short stature have as many problems from twenty to thirty pounds of overweight as taller people have from more.

Total fasting is so treacherous, even in the best of hands, that the *modified fast* was introduced. The rice diet (see page 97) is one type of modified fast. This diet gives just enough calories to fend off ketosis.

The 500-calorie diet is another modified fast. A typical 500-calorie diet would be: one hard-cooked egg, one glass of nonfat milk, a large salad with diet dressing or no dressing, and one or two pieces of very low density fruit. This is the *total* day's food. Many people regularly put themselves on a modified fast such as the 500-calorie diet to lose a few pounds gained by too much partying.

The protein-sparing modified fast has no advantage over the simple 500-calorie diet given above. Too much protein potentially increases the work the kidneys have to do.

If you are not pregnant and have no health problems—no tendency to anorexia nervosa or hair loss—the 500-calorie, simple diet is harmless. If you have little weight to lose (under fifteen to twenty pounds) and do not need to learn new food or eating habits, the simple 500-calorie modified fast is fine.

Hair loss is, however, not uncommon when daily calorie intake drops this low. Some people who go on very low-calorie crash diets to lose twenty or more pounds fast, lose all their hair. Even though the hair grows back in time, if you have a susceptibility to hair loss, a crash diet may bring out the tendency.

Complete loss of hair has occurred in people who have had expensive hair transplants. And transplanted hair, once lost, does *not* grow back. A crash diet can act as an experiment on your hair. You have to decide whether it is worth the risk.

How successful is medically supervised fasting for more serious weight problems—for people with more than twenty pounds to lose? The answer depends entirely on the individual. If you daydream about a future filled with whipped cream and chocolates, steak and crullers, your chances of gaining the weight back are good.

If you can get your mind on things other than food and determine to be satisfied with a future where you eat to live instead of live to eat, your fasting will not be in vain.

Here is a review of the diets that are making fasting a fad.

TABLE 5. FASTS AND MODIFIED FASTS

Title	Chief Characteristics
Fasting: The Ultimate Diet Cott	The author is reassuring about the ease, safety, and advantages of fasting. Although book advises medical supervision, it is likely that many people, especially moderately overweight people, will be motivated to fast on their own. Young people who are subject to anorexia nervosa can be greatly harmed by the stimulating emotional effects of quick weight loss and loss of appetite, both caused by ketosis. The harm to these and other people comes from prolonged fasting which is encouraged by the effects of ketosis. "Long-term problems of prolonged fasting, significant, but initially less dramatic, would be created by the great loss of protein from vital tissues and the mineral losses from skeletal and soft tissues," according to Dr. Philip L. White, Director, AMA Department of Foods and Nutrition. In spite of reassurances in this book, the consensus of the most concerned medical specialists is that total fasting for more than a day or two is not recommended without hospitalization. There are too many things that can go wrong. People with diabetes, a tendency toward hypoglycemia, heart disease, or stroke should never fast except under strict medical guidance. Pregnant women should never fast. Frequent monitoring of various chemical components of the blood is necessary during fasts of more than a day or two. People who have no reason to believe they have gout or anemia, for example, have gotten these conditions during prolonged fasting. People who are in hazardous occupations should not fast. Driving a car is hazardous and nutritionist Dr. White advises that fasting with its attendant low blood pressure, weakness, nausea, and light headedness makes driving even more hazardous.
Protein-Sparing Modified Fast: PSMF Blackburn, Genuth	The PSMF consists of no food except 250 to 500 calories daily of a protein supplement. Total fasting causes considerable loss of body protein as well as body fat. Body protein is spared by the small amount of calories in this diet. A relatively small amount of carbohydrate also spares body protein (see rice diet, page 97). However, the name PSMF is used for the

protein supplement diet. The protein supplement consists of pre-digested animal protein made into amino acids by industrial chemical methods. While the PSMF is of scientific and experimental interest, its potential for both good and harm has by no means been entirely worked out. Pure amino acid diets are ketogenic (see page 87). Many long-range problems associated with ketogenic diets, such as the loss of calcium from bones and the connection of this loss to aging, require more scientific study. Many people are endangered by the immediate effects of ketogenic diets. Some of the scientific study-diets have enough added glucose to prevent the PSMF from being ketogenic. Dr. George L. Blackburn from the Department of Surgery at Harvard University Medical school, one of the principal investigators of the PSMF, points out that the use of this diet for obesity is in its experimental stages.

Dr. Linn's Last Chance Diet
Linn

Advocates the PSMF and suggests the use of Prolinn, an amino acid mixture colored and flavored with cherry juice. Prolinn has the same amino acid composition as another product (E.M.F.). Several similar products are flavored with orange, lemon, or cherry juice. The amino acid mixtures used in these products differ from some of the scientific investigations of the PSMF.* Author Linn's suggested daily dose of Prolinn is 4 to 5 ounces per day for women and 7 to 8 ounces per day for men. Pre-digested animal collagen products usually contain 15 grams of protein per ounce (60 calories), as does Prolinn. Although author states there are no major side effects, his readers are warned to have uric acid checked and to be guided by a doctor. The appetite-decreasing effect of this ketogenic diet is described as beneficial. Book advises what to do for obvious unpleasant effects of ketosis: bad breath, fatigue, nausea, cramps in arms and legs. Author Linn also advises that intestinal gas from a no-fiber diet is not serious. Return-to-eating diet is a version of the exchange diet (see page 217). Vitamin pills, water, coffee, tea, or diet soda, moderate exercise and behavior modification, are advocated.

*Pre-digested protein products (e.g., Prolinn, E.M.F., T-Amino, Amino-Sol, Pro-Fast) are made from animal collagens. Some sources of animal collagens are animal hoofs and skins. Some of the scientific studies have been done using animal collagen products, others have used milk protein (casein), unprocessed meat such as steak, egg white, or soy protein. The significance of this difference to the people on these diets is not known.

LOW-CALORIE BALANCED DIETS

Doctors have been handing out low-calorie balanced diets for years. You've probably had a few given to you. *The diets work. But they don't solve the weight problem.* Why not?

You and millions of other people started dieting for a few days in good faith. Then your commitment failed. It takes at least as long to get rid of overweight as it takes to put it on. It's only human to want something fast and easy.

You could never find a satisfactory way to reinforce your commitment. Pills made you sick or high. Foods that urge you to eat more got in your way.

And the fact is that if you could keep to the small portions of food on these diets, you wouldn't have had a weight problem in the first place.

I want to show you some other things about low-calorie balanced diets to help you understand that the key to losing weight is realizing that *no single diet is good for everybody.*

First, let's talk about balancing.

What Is a Balanced Diet?

The old notion of a balanced diet is based on the average North American way of eating. This is typically:

>   50 percent carbohydrate
>   20 percent protein
>   30 percent fat

Let's take 1,200 calories.

The average North American woman will lose weight on 1,200 calories a day and maintain a new low weight on 1,400 to 1,600 calories. The average North American man will lose weight on 1,500 calories a day and maintain a new weight on 1,800 to 2,000 calories.

Let's translate percentages of the major food groups into weights and portion sizes: First is carbohydrate: 600 calories, or 50 percent of 1,200, is first divided by four, the calories per gram of carbohydrates. This is 150 grams. And 150 grams of carbohydrate is:

>   Two and three-fourths cups of dry oatmeal, or eight and one-third ounces by weight, which will cook up into between eight and nine cups because

you add water. This is a little over eight times more than the usual portion, which is one ounce by weight or one-third cup by volume. It is important to remember that there are also forty-one-and-a-half grams of protein in two and three-fourths cups of dry oatmeal as well as 150 grams of carbohydrate.

4–9 slices of bread, depending on the size of the slices and the type of bread
9 medium-sized baked or boiled potatoes with the skins
4–5 whole medium-sized canteloupes
7–8 whole grapefruits

Now, let's take protein: 240 calories, or 20 percent of 1,200, is first divided by four, the calories per gram of protein. Each of the following amounts of food represents 60 grams of protein:

9 pieces of plain poached or broiled fish, without any fat or skin. Each piece is 2 inches square and 1 inch thick, pressed into tablespoons gives 16
8 pieces of any meat (beef, lamb, pork, liver, chicken, or turkey) very lean, very well trimmed. Each piece is 2 inches long by 2 inches wide by ¼ inch thick
25 small, 10 medium, or 4½ large sardines without any added fat
8 thin slices of cheddar cheese (8 ounces)
10½ ounces of non-fat cottage cheese. You will exceed your daily allowance of fat calories if you eat the equivalent of 60 grams of protein in creamed cottage cheese.
9 large eggs or 11½ small eggs will give you 60 grams of protein, but you will exceed your daily fat calories.
6 ounces of peanut butter or 12 tablespoons will give you 60 grams of protein, but you will exceed your daily fat allowance by double. Peanut butter is a food to break the rules with for weight-conscious people.

Now, let's take fat: 360 calories or 30 percent of 1,200 is divided by nine, the calories per gram of fat. This is 40 grams of fat. *Note that you already have 40 grams of fat or even much more from your protein food. You already have about 5 grams of fat from your carbohydrate food, unless you chose plain potato, rice, beans, corn, or oats without any fat mixed in.*

In other words, the popular American protein foods bring so much fat along with them that you can't eat very much food without getting too much fat and far too many calories.

Nevertheless, let's take a look at the amounts of some popular fatty foods that contain 40 grams of fat:

3½ well-done, crisp slices of bacon
8 teaspoons of mayonnaise, oil, margarine, butter, or solid cooking fat (lard or vegetable-oil shortening)

8 tablespoons of heavy cream, sour cream, or sour cream substitute
14 tablespoons of light cream
7 tablespoons of cream cheese
40 small olives
45 small nuts (approximately)

Problems with Low-Calorie Balanced Diets

The problem with low-calorie balanced diets is that you do not get very much to eat. You can have four small servings of plain, mainly starchy foods: bread, crackers, rice, potato, cereal. You can have five small servings of mainly protein food: fish, egg, meat, poultry, or cheese. You can have three small pieces of fruit, one small serving of cooked medium-starch vegetable such as beets, carrots, onions, peas, or squash, as much raw green vegetable as· you want, a scant one-eighth portion of any of the things on the list of popular fatty foods, and eight ounces of milk (preferably nonfat for everybody with diabetes, coronary disease, and gall bladder disease in their genetic programming).

Overall, the volume of food is small; it might begin to satisfy you after six months to a year or more of working on your will to learn to have a smaller appetite. If you have a big appetite, you will still be hungry after a day of 1,200 calories eaten this way unless you choose low-density foods.

You can tell from the quantities given how small the portions have to be. If you increase portion sizes just a little, there is a significant increase in calories. (Note that in the foods listed above, cantaloupe and grapefruit are very low density carbohydrates.) If you eat just a little of foods that urge you to eat more, page 8, there is significant increase in calories.

Another problem with these diets is that they contain too much saturated fat, especially for people who have a genetic weakness for cholesterol diseases.

The newer trend in diet balancing is 30 percent protein and 20 percent fat. Even with this change, saturated fat is too high for many people because saturated fats account for almost half of the composition of most meats.

These facts about diet balancing are important, but even more important is that *everybody's need for each of the three major food groups is different* (see Chapter 9, "Nutrition Facts for Overweight People"). You have to work out your own needs. They are part of your appetite pattern. *And remember, being hungry is the best way to wreck a weight-loss program.*

The next thing you need to know is how much of each of the three major food groups you should have for good health. You will want to know what actual foods will supply your health needs and best fit your tastes.

Following is a survey of low-calorie balanced diets. There are many others—versions of either the "prudent diet" or "exchange system." Often, you will find mixtures of them with a twist of some kind—add physical exercise; add fasting somewhere along the line; add mental, emotional, or mystical supports; add group help.

You will notice that each of the diets surveyed here tries to catch your fancy by using a famous name or some other trick.

TABLE 6. LOW-CALORIE BALANCED DIETS*

Title	Chief Characteristics
Exchange Diet, developed through joint efforts of the American Diabetes Association and American Medical Association Department of Nutrition	All standard American foods divided into seven basic lists; the only sucrose-containing foods are plain sponge cake and vanilla ice cream, intended as treats for special occasions as this diet was originally prepared for sugar-sensitive people. *Excellent method for all interested people to become knowledgeable in fundamentals of nutrition by comparing equivalent foods all of which contain the same nutrient components.* Also useful for people who wish to choose highest volume of food with least food energy since dimensions and weight are given for each item; you pick your own foods from the exchange lists, based on how many calories per day you desire, and according to your personal needs for the basic food groups. The average woman will lose fat at 1,200 calories per day and the average man at approximately 1,500 calories. You can add calories of food to *make up* for extra output from exercise or heavy work. Notice that portion sizes are small, and that binges are only allowed from List 1 (see pages 217–221 for the Original Exchange Diet). The exchange diet is the model that all low-calorie balanced diets are patterned after.
Workingman's Diet	Very low in calories—700—balanced in the three major groups; recommends a little lower fat than so-called American average—about 20 percent fat and 30 percent protein. Other than this, recommends an initial fast of two days, which is controversial due to potential for ketosis.
New You Diet	1,200-calorie diet, gives you seven days of menus—to take the need to think out of dieting. Advocates long daily walks and relaxation.
Mademoiselle Editor's Diet	Low-calorie balanced diet plus nibbling of low-calorie food.

*50 percent carbohydrate, 20 percent protein, 30 percent fat.

Astronaut's Diet (also known as Dr. Smith's Astronaut's Diet)	The exchange diet with lists of low-cholesterol foods—some of which are disputed and controversial according to American Heart Association recommendations.
The Prudent Man's Diet Jolliffe	There are many later versions of this approach, some unchanged, others changed slightly. Dr. Norman Jolliffe was for many years head of the Nutrition Bureau, New York City Health Department. This is a 2,400 calorie, low-saturated fat, low-cholesterol, low-salt diet; 2,400 calories is too high for most sedentary American adults.
Prudent Diet Bennett and Simon	Follows Jolliffe's example, but a little lower in total fat, a little higher in protein; low in refined carbohydrate and salt. By the most up to date criteria, there is too much fat.
You Can Do It Proxmire	Senator William Proxmire, an ardent advocate of good health and nutrition in the U.S. Senate and lifetime calorie-watcher presents his low-calorie balanced diet and discusses some of his personal food binges with calorie counts of food energy amounting to up to 1,700 calories for a single binge.
Wise Woman's Diet Redbook magazine, put together for Redbook by George Christakis, M.D., who worked with Dr. Jolliffe	Change in gender from Prudent Man's Diet; fat increased by 3 percent.
But I Don't Eat That Much Glenn	Dr. M. B. Glenn, also a former colleague of Dr. Jolliffe's, presents a selection of Prudent Diet plans—you pick your diet according to your sex, your activity, and how much you weigh.
Easy, No-Risk Diet Solomon and Sheppard	This is a version of the exchange diet; no discussion of fat, and saturated fat is high just as in the original; the idea here is that you don't have to count up calories—the diet does it for you.
Mayo Clinic Diet Mayo Clinic Diet Manual	The original—and there are many fakes that try to cash in on the name of the Mayo Clinic. This is the exchange diet with an extensive nomogram version of standard height and weight charts. From the Mayo Clinic Diet Manual used by the Clinic in the dietary department.
Weight Watchers	Basically a version of the prudent diet, with addition of group-psychology method; originally, WW shunned diet foods, but now has a big line of frozen and ordinary shelf items competing with the rest of the commercial brands (see page 113).
One Day at a Time Small	A low-calorie (1,200 a day) balanced diet, with the twist that obesity is like alcoholism, but the addiction is to food; basically a version of the prudent diet with an Alcoholics Anonymous platform.
Ladies' Home Journal Family Diet Book	A composite of all the prudent diets and the exchange diet; 1,200 calories; the portion sizes are explicitly spelled out and are small; it tells you how many "food

units" you can take from each food group so that you can make accurate exchanges.

The Computer Diet	Computer-compiled lists and charts so you can select your own diet based on how much you want to lose.
Cadence Nutritional Diets	There are several mail-order versions of computer diets. You fill out a lengthy form and mail it to the service. The computer picks out your diet, in the form of printouts of menus.

GIMMICK DIETS

The oldest and most harmful gimmick "diet" cannot possibly rise up to harm you. The gimmick consisted of a tapeworm pressed into a tablet. The first Pure Food and Drug Laws passed in the early 1900s put an end to this gimmick version of *eat all you want.*

The more recent gimmick diets make use of prayer, self-hypnosis, even sex (note the Lover's Diet). The gimmick gets the emphasis. You aren't supposed to notice that the food part of the diet is an ordinary low-calorie balanced diet. Gimmick diets are blindfolds, and the harm they do is that they confuse you.

Any method that gives you the idea that it works by some magic trick makes you dependent on tricks and gimmicks. You have to strip the window dressing and fancy packaging from these methods and see what makes them tick; then you are independent.

Look over the gimmick diets here.

TABLE 7. GIMMICK DIETS

Title	Chief Characteristics
Candy Diet	Ayds, and so on. The idea is that one or two candies with 25 calories of food energy before each meal depresses appetite, allowing you to eat *small helpings* rather than big helpings. Comment: "They didn't depress mine"—Peter Wyden in *Overweight Society.*
Lover's Diet Friedman	A single act of sexual intercourse burns an average of 400 calories/hour for a 150 pound person* Also avoid sweets and fats, but mainly reach for a mate instead of a plate.
Nibbler's Diet	This is the frequent-small-meal idea, which is more than a gimmick as nibbling helps satisfy some people.

*Smaller people will burn fewer calories, larger people will burn more. Sexual intercourse is a 5–6 MET activity.

	However, the theory that this eating style *depletes* fat storage is a gimmick and has been disproven; only fewer total calories of food energy taken in than energy plus heat put out depletes fat storage. It is important, therefore, to count all your calories for the day.
Temptation Diet	A form of aversion or revulsion therapy; you eat one tempting food until you're sick of it; another way to aversion is to eat in some circumstance that is disgusting, revolting, or horrifying to you.
Diet through Sleep	A mail-order send-in-the-coupon gimmick that reappears from time to time. Another approach to mind-over-matter emphasizing self-discipline to help you stick out a low-calorie diet; recommends relaxation and self-hypnosis or autosuggestion; for example, at bedtime, repeat to yourself: "I am growing thinner and thinner."
Expense Account Diet	Instead of a high-calorie, high-density hotdog or hamburger for lunch, go to an expensive restaurant and order gourmet dishes but *without* sauces and be sure they are foods you know are low or relatively low in fat and low in calories. Dine slowly while satisfying yourself more on service and atmosphere than on food.
The Fat Is in Your Head Rev. Charlie W. Shedd	Mind-over-matter method for persons who follow religion and praying as part of their life style. Author features prayer against weight and has had a number of books. This one adds behavior modification.

HIGH-FIBER DIETS

Unfortunately, there is no miracle diet that will melt fat, lower blood cholesterol, and solve all your problems.

Not even the high-fiber diet will do all these things.

The story behind the high-fiber diet starts with an English doctor who studied diseases of African village people who had moved to the city. The doctor concluded that when these people gave up the bran they ate in the villages and switched to refined flour and sugar, they began to have constipation, which is common in countries like the United States and Canada.

Out of this observation, there grew all sorts of speculation about what bran *might do.*

By now, scientific studies have turned in lots of data about what bran does and doesn't do.

What Does Bran Do?

Bran is very helpful for relieving constipation. There isn't anything new about that.

Bran does this by leaving fiber in the gastrointestinal tract. The fiber isn't absorbed into the body's bloodstream. It doesn't get into the metabolic systems.

This leftover fiber increases the bulkiness of the stool. Bulkiness counteracts constipation.

Is Leftover Fiber Unique to Bran?

Bran is far from being the only food that can provide fiber in our diets. The other fiber-containing foods are more suitable for overweight people because they are more filling and satisfying. (You will find more information about food fiber in Chapter 9, on page 145, and a list of fiber-containing foods on page 203.)

Note that diseases of the large intestine such as colitis and diverticulitis can get worse from too much bran consumption.

How Much Bran Is Too Much?

This is an individual matter. Bloating, gas, cramping or pain from eating bran needs to be checked out by a doctor. Bran can cause irritation in the bowel. Corn, nuts, and small seeds from berries can also irritate the bowel when people have colitis and diverticulitis.

Serious trouble such as peritonitis occasionally comes on from too much irritation.

Large amounts of bran block the absorption of iron from the gastrointestinal tract. This is due to a substance in bran called *phytic acid* that combines with the food iron and forces it into the waste products in the bowel. Many overweight people in North America are low in iron and are anemic. Between 20 and 50 percent of North American girls between seventeen and nineteen years of age are anemic. Loss of food iron is unfortunate for these people.

Phytic acid also decreases absorption of calcium from the gastrointestinal tract.

In a whole loaf of whole-wheat bread you get the same amount of phytic acid as you get from two teaspoonfuls of bran after each meal. It's much healthier to eat bran spread out in the form of whole wheat. There have been a number of studies on whether high-bran diets will lower blood cholesterol. Cholesterol lowering by bran is not proven.

It's not what you eat that lowers blood cholesterol. It's not what you eat that gets the fat out of your system. *It's what you don't eat that does these things.* You can't eat all you want of high-fat foods and expect a big dose of bran to get rid of the consequences.

The highlights of the high-fiber fad diets are covered here so that you will be familiar with them:

TABLE 8. HIGH-FIBER DIETS

Title	Chief Characteristics
High Fiber Diet Fredericks Rubin	Originally suggested by Burkitt in England and popularized in several versions in the United States. Low-calorie, high-fiber, and roughage, some meat. Advocates large amounts of bran flakes, which may be irritating to susceptible people who have gastrointestinal problems. Because of phytic acid in bran, blockage of iron absorption may cause or aggravate iron-deficiency anemia in susceptible people. Advocates honey or molasses for sweeteners—*these are the same chemical ingredients as sucrose.* In theory, the "back fifty to one hundred years diet" idea is good, but large amounts of bran have caused intestinal obstruction, cramps, gas, and abdominal distention in many people.

WHAT HAVE WE LEARNED FROM FAD DIETS?

You should start thinking of the word *diet* as a total approach to eating to live—not as a crash or fad experiment on your body.

Every person has an individual set of inherited and noninherited food and nutritional needs. No single diet is best for everybody.

The long-range health and preventive-medicine prediction for the future calls for individual lifetime diet prescriptions from the time of birth.

Moderation in all things relating to food and exercise is the key to lifetime weight control.

FACTS ABOUT DIET FOODS

What do we mean by diet foods?

Powdered nonfat milk is a good diet food. A fresh pear or a whole baked potato eaten with the skin is a good diet food. Raw carrots are a good diet food. All these foods have fine nutritional ingredients and are low in calories for the bulk, or volume, of food that you eat. But these foods are not usually thought of as diet foods.

The term "diet food" is generally used for a commercial preparation. The words "diet food" give the illusion that the product is low-calorie.

Commercial diet foods fall into seven general categories. Viewing them this way helps you to see through the illusions.

Prepared Diet Food

Diet cookies, candy, and desserts are usually sweetened in part artificially and contain only a few less calories than the real thing. These foods are usually still high in fat.

Diet syrups, jams, jellies, gelatin desserts, and stewed fruits are artificially sweetened. They are harmless in moderate amounts, if you must have sweets other than fresh fruit.

So-called diet dinners and portions of food are usually frozen. These products do not have significantly fewer calories than ordinary preparations of the same things.

Diet bars contain a calorie-counted sweetened mixture of chocolate and milk products. These are high in processed sugar and are not sensible foods. For 250 calories, you can have an apple, a piece of low-fat cheese, and a slice of whole-wheat bread. You not only have to eat refined sugar in the diet bar but you get no trace minerals.

Diet Beverages

Diet soda contains as much phosphorus as regular sugar-sweetened soda.

Excess phophorous pulls calcium out of bones. Diet soda also contains a large amount of salt. Read the contents on the label of the soda can. You will see that there are a number of sodium compounds in the diet drink. Your body retains water from any sodium compound, not just table salt. Remember that *sodium* gave the name *soda* to these drinks.

Nonfat milk drinks, artificially sweetened and flavored, are a compromise for rare occasions. In moderation, they are harmless.

Low-calorie presweetened tea is another compromise for special occasions. There is a suggestion for decreasing the amount of sweetener in presweetened tea on pages 164–165.

Artificial Sweeteners*

There will always be a safe, noncaloric sweetener on the market. The chief problem with these sweeteners is that they feed your sweet tooth. And they don't free your spirit to assert itself against sweets. When you feel you have to have a sweet drink, artificially sweetened tea, coffee, lemonade, and milk are safe compromises. Remember that moderate quantities of all foods and beverages are best.

Salt Substitutes

These are usually potassium or half-and-half sodium and potassium (see page 32). They are safe in small amounts. First try to get over your taste for excessive amounts of salt; then a little salt substitute is usually harmless for most people.

Low-Fat Processed Dairy Products

Although they are highly processed, they have a place. Remember, there is still fat remaining; use them in moderation. Lite-Line™ produces both cream cheese and American cheese foods that contain 30 percent less fat than the usual versions.

---

*In March 1977 two newspaper stories appeared. One referred to the FDA ban on saccharin. The other referred to a new natural sweetener, either low calorie or noncaloric, derived from citrus fruit peel. The scientific and human-use evidence to date indicates that saccharin, and cyclamates, are probably not harmful in moderate amounts. Nevertheless, bans on artificial sweeteners may serve as motivation for further research on safe, noncaloric sweeteners from natural sources.

Imitation Mayonnaise

This product contains 50 percent less fat than ordinary mayonnaise. Try to break the mayonnaise habit. You don't need it. But if you must have mayonnaise at times, this imitation is a good compromise. Common sense says to use very small amounts.

Diet Salad Dressings

Read the label. These products have less oil than regular dressings, sometimes no oil. Try to break the habit for heavily sweetened condiments, but a little diet salad dressing can make the lettuce easy to eat, and that is helpful. There is a suggestion for lowering the salt and calories of processed diet salad dressings on page 181.

Miracle Remedies— Fact or Fiction?

7

TRICKS AND RIPOFFS

There are two inexpensive, plain, undramatic, sure ways to weight control: a lifetime of suitable personal eating and a lifetime of suitable personal body activity.

Yet a ten-billion-dollar-a-year weight-control industry is thriving in North America. Our weight-conscious think-thin society provides a steady market for everything from fad diets to dangerous surgery and "zippers for the mouth."

It's only human to want a quick, effortless, and magical way to reach a difficult goal. It is so human that the United States Food and Drug Administration and its counterpart in Canada can't stay abreast of the tricks and ripoffs that keep appearing in the weight-control industry.

Remember that the power of the Food and Drug Administration and the Federal Trade Commission is defined within strict and narrow guidelines. The usual advertising tactic of diet-and-exercise gimmicks is the offer of an *illusion* of relief from your problem. As long as no harm from the gimmick can be proven, the FDA has no case.

The Federal Trade Commission and the Canadian Consumer Protection Board have made an issue of deceptive advertising and pricing. When advertising promises weight loss and quick, lasting results, they have grounds to charge deception.

For example, in *Gloria Marshall Figure Control Salons* vs. *The Federal Trade Commission,* the regulatory agency charged that the ads made false promises. The ads promised free figure analysis, a half-hour treatment for two dollars and fifty cents, and "quick, lasting results." The FTC said that customers were "exposed to sales pitches for expensive health and weight programs," and weight loss couldn't last "without dietary restriction." The FTC also alleged that instead of paying two dollars and fifty cents for each treatment, customers were required to buy 140 treatments.

The ads that had been placed in Indianapolis newspapers were withdrawn.

Recently, the U.S. Congress voted to give the Food and Drug Administration increased authority to protect consumers from items considered by a panel of authorities to be health hazards. But that protection isn't the whole answer. You also have to have the inner strength and knowledge to protect yourself against things that are harmless and also useless.

Rolling and Massage

Rolling and massage by human hands or with the aid of a mechanical device are as old as history. In 1964 the Federal Trade Commission put a stop to an electrically operated oscillating table sold under the name of the Stauffer Home Reducing Plan. The feature of the plan was a "magic couch, the famous Posture Rest." The FTC found that Stauffer Laboratories, Inc., "advertised effortless exercise and calorie reduction." The regulatory action put a stop to the false and deceptive advertising, but this was not possible until hundreds of thousands of public dollars had been spent by the regulators. How much consumer money was spent is not known.

The Relaxacizor, an electrical device, was said to be effective for waistline reducing by providing electrical shocks to the body. Electrical shocks cause muscle contractions. In this way the device was supposed to be similar to massage. In 1970 a United States District Court agreed with the Food and Drug Administration that the device was harmful and issued a permanent injunction prohibiting the sale of the Relaxacizor. "There is a wide spectrum of conditions in which the Relaxacizor is hazardous and contraindicated," the Judge of the United States District Court said in his opinion. The Court found that this device may cause a miscarriage and may aggravate a number of conditions such as epilepsy, hernia, ulcers, and varicose veins. The distributor, Relaxacizor, Inc., appealed, but the appeal was dismissed.

What is massaging, and what does it do? Massaging is passive exercise, in contrast to active exercise, which is done by your own muscles. Passive exercise helps you feel good—a worthwhile goal, but you don't burn energy from rolling, tilting, vibrating, or being massaged. You cannot lose weight when you don't burn energy.

Gyms, where active exercise is pursued, may use overkill advertising techniques, but exercise is exercise. Whether it's done at home, at a gym, at a park, or someplace else, the ground rules for active exercise and calorie loss hold good (see page 34).

In the case of passive exercise, the masseuse or masseur does the work and burns up the calories.

What about an expensive little block of plastic called a "Five Minute Waist Slimmer"? As with any massaging device, you might just as well use your hands. If you massage yourself, with your hands or with a device, you will burn a small amount of energy, but not enough to lose weight.

Belts, Girdles, and Plastic Wrappings

These devices accomplish the same thing as massage.

The Federal Trade Commission restrained the sale of "exercise belts" because of misleading advertising. But the belts have returned to the market under a new guise. They have appeared as outer wear and feature a buckle with a buzz. The buzzing buckle is supposed to remind you to pull your *tummy* in. There's no false advertising, only the appeal of the illusion of slimness for people who can't remember to pull in their tummies.

Lifetime programs of right eating and exercise are surer and healthier ways of getting your *tummy down and in.*

Flab—or cellulite, if you prefer—is easy to mold or compress by a girdle or a wrapping into something that *looks better* for a short time.

But you don't expend energy, you don't burn calories, and the compression *wears off* in a day or two and you have accomplished nothing.

Cellulite is described as a combination of "fat, water, and wastes trapped in lumpy, immovable pockets just beneath the skin" by a nonmedical French writer Nicole Ronsard. "It is those jodhpur thighs, saddleback buttocks or bumpy looking legs that remind you of cottage cheese or knees that seem full of little bumps."

This description fits the facts about fatty tissue emptied of triglyceride and partly filled with body water (see page 24).

Wrapping and massaging the flab helps, but only for a short time. This external pressure gives only temporary improvement to the body's outward appearance because it compresses the cells so they are closer together. But they soon spread again.

Ronsard's diet no-no's are sensible because they are high-fat foods (peanut butter, sour cream, bacon, TV dinners), high-fat and high-sugar combinations (malts, shakes), and high-salt foods (TV dinners, canned soups, bouillon cubes, bacon).

Sweat Inducers

When you sweat without your body having to *work* for it, you will lose only water weight. You won't even lose water trapped inside half-empty fat cells.

The water you lose is the important water in your bloodstream.

This is why saunas and sweat suits can be dangerous.

Either of these sweating methods can cause sudden, rapid dehydration. The human body reacts very quickly to fast water loss. Rapid dehydration is stressful. It brings on the adrenalin-stress response.

Water loss from the blood makes the blood thicker and stickier. A big slug of adrenalin and sticky blood are set-ups for a coronary occlusion in susceptible people with cholesterol plaques.

Danger is not the only drawback to sweating for weight loss.

The heat loss from your body is slowed way down because internal body heat loss is less in a hot environment. Remember how that heat loss, especially after a meal, helps you lose calories?

You can see how sweating without exercising defeats your purpose.

Exercise Devices

The illusion of quickie body shaping is very appealing. But there's nothing a pushing-and-pulling gadget will do except isometric exercises.

Anybody can do isometric exercises without any gadget whatsoever.

Isometric exercises burn few calories and, because they make the heart work up against a resistance, they elevate blood pressure.

Working against a resistance is like banging against a steel wall or trying to fight City Hall.

The small number of calories burned and the danger to people with hypertension are not the only drawbacks to exercise gadgets.

Gadgets get between you and your will power.

They build up an illusion that something magic outside yourself will take away your overweight.

Only your body can take in energy and only your body can put energy out.

Self-Hypnosis—Disguised

Have you ever seen big ads that tell you: "Your fat will melt away while you sleep"?

You send off for the mail-order treatment and it turns out to be lessons in self-hypnosis and instructions for exercise and a low-calorie balanced diet.

There is nothing wrong with exercise and a low-calorie balanced diet.

It's the ad that's misleading. The ad is deceptive and uses the technique of *illusion.*

PARAMEDICAL AND MEDICAL TREATMENTS

Acupuncture, BBs and Earrings

Acupuncture consists of sticking needles into the skin at certain "points." There is a "point" for appetite control in the ear.

Earrings, BBs, and other devices taped onto an earlobe are supposed to remind you to change old bad food and eating habits for new good ones. A staple or decorative needle in the ear at the acupuncture "point" is supposed to have the same effect.

A large amount of objective research has been done in the United States on how acupuncture works. The results indicate that it works on the mind —and is similar to self-hypnosis. Ear devices become a middleman between yourself and your will power.

Your self-control will be stronger if you don't have a go-between attached to it. Besides, you can take your self-control with you everywhere you go. It goes to parties and socials with you; it goes to weddings and buffets.

What's more, at home, especially when you're alone, your self-control is all you have. Your goal is to be independent and free of eating problems. The key to independence is self-contained; it is inside yourself—your will power.

Biofeedback and Aversion Therapy

In biofeedback, the patient is hooked up to a machine. A therapist talks to the patient about appetite, food, and eating habits. When the patient makes the right responses, for example, "I will stop eating pizza and ice cream after dinner," the therapist has the machine make pleasant sounds. When the patient says the wrong words, for example, "I hardly eat a thing," the therapist has the machine make unpleasant sounds. The memories of the sounds are supposed to be recalled when the patient has trouble with food and eating situations in everyday life.

This may sound like a simplified explanation for a seemingly complex process. The important fact, however, is that you become dependent on a machine to strengthen your mind. Remember that your goal must be total independence. Dependency on a machine or a device as a go-between is not enough.

Aversion is another method. A therapist gives a small electric shock to a patient while the conversation covers bad eating habits.

Another kind of aversion therapy associates bad smells or tastes with food and eating.

Both of these methods depend on outside devices—a machine, a shock, a bad taste or odor.

Outside devices tend to fog up the facts. They give you the idea that a magic trick will solve your problem. You forget that your mind and your will have to be independent twenty-four hours a day. Independence and maturity are your keys to success. You need to have all your forces within yourself for maximum success.

A Zipper on Your Mouth

Have you ever wished you could put a zipper on your mouth? This is what the jaw-wiring operation tries to accomplish. A dentist has to wire the jaws together and then later remove the wires. So, you see, it's not as simple as a zipper on your jacket or pants.

While the wires are in place, it's impossible to eat solid food. All nourishment has to be liquid and taken with a straw. Several people have choked to death when they got sick and vomited.

For others, the lifetime results are poor. After the wires are removed, nearly everyone gains back the weight lost while the jaws were wired.

These people have centered their whole attention on weight loss. They haven't learned the necessary lessons about how to eat to maintain weight loss.

Health Spas, Fat Farms, Fat Camps, and Reducing Gyms

All these establishments are in business to help you lose weight with the aid of exercise.

In theory, this is a noble pursuit.

Exercise is good for weight loss no matter where you go to do it.

Millions of North Americans are turning to exercise, and the health-spa business is booming. The Federal Trade Commission and the Canadian Consumer Protection Board report that the complaints are also booming.

One of the problems that these regulatory bodies have run into is in how to define these businesses. In the end, the definition came out as "Services or facilities to improve physical condition or appearance through change in weight, weight control, treatment, dieting or exercise."

The definition of a health spa used by the Association of Physical Fitness Centers is a little different from the Federal Trade Commission's definition. The Association says a health spa is a place offering a "contract for instruction, training or assistance in physical culture, exercising, reducing, physical development or any other such activity or for the use of the facilities of a health spa or gymnasium used for any of the above purposes."

The word "contract" is the source of most complaints about gyms and spas. Short-term contracts, usually offered at special rates, cause the bulk of the complaints.

Consumers complain to the regulatory bodies that they didn't lose the weight the ad promised. People complain that they weren't told they had to change eating habits and sign up for much longer terms of exercise than the original contract called for.

This is how spas and gyms have gotten a reputation for using illusory and deceptive advertising called *bait-and-switch methods.*

Be sure you know exactly what you're getting and what facilities will be available. Make sure you know and are satisfied with the hours the gym or spa is open before you sign anything.

All the spas and gyms that have sprung up in the big cities are *not* given to use of false advertising. The well-run establishments serve a need by providing heated indoor swimming pools and exercise facilities for people who have no other place for these activities. They also fill a need for people who are embarrassed to be seen exercising out of doors in public view.

Another kind of facility is a sleepover spa, called a "fat farm" for adults or a "fat camp" for children and teenagers.

Fat camps for overweight children and adolescents fail unless they make every effort to teach the youngsters *new* exercise and eating habits.

Children generally lose weight at any camp. Then they go home, back to their old food and eating habits, and regain the weight. The yo-yo syndrome can start at a very young age.

Many overweight youngsters are too embarrassed to exercise in the city. Unless a fat camp can get a young person to exercise all year round, it is no better than an ordinary camp.

Many adults prefer to spend their vacations at "fat farms" instead of resorts. But the lifetime results aren't very good when you consider how many people regain the weight they lost.

PILLS AND POTENT MEDICATIONS

Nonprescription medicine for sale over the counter or by mail order is now limited to things that will do no harm.

What is meant by *no harm?*

Even aspirin is harmful in susceptible people.

Amphetamines, such as Benzedrine and Dexedrine, decrease appetite in some people, but not in everybody. They are now sold only by prescription, since it has been proven that they can cause addiction.

Hormones, especially thyroid, do nothing for overweight except in very high, dangerous doses.

Digitalis, a potent heart drug, makes you lose your appetite and get sick to your stomach.

It's hard to believe that these potent medicines were so easy to obtain till very recently.

A combination of these three drugs, amphetamine, thyroid, and digitalis, used to be sold by weight specialists. The drug combinations were put in bright-colored capsules and were called *rainbow pills.* The amphetamine part of the pills was supposed to decrease appetite; the thyroid part was supposed to increase the metabolic rate; the digitalis part made people sick to their stomachs.

The capsules were banned after a number of deaths of people who had been taking them resulted in a United States Senate investigation (Diet Pill Industry Hearings Before the Subcommittee on Antitrust and Monopoly, 90th Congress, 1968).

What kinds of pills and medicines can you still buy on your own?

Methyl cellulose is an old-timer in weight control. It is a chemically purified component of the pulp of fruits and vegetables. Methyl cellulose swells up into a large bulk when it's mixed with water.

Methyl cellulose is also sold in tablet form or in a wafer that looks like a small graham cracker.

Concentrated methyl cellulose is known to cause obstruction plugs in the intestinal tract. These require surgery for removal.

It's far safer to eat cellulose in the natural form of vegetables and fruits, where you get your cellulose mixed with minerals, trace minerals, and vitamins. You also get it mixed with natural amounts of water.

Mild diuretics are another type of over-the-counter weight-reducing medicine. The diuretics are combined with a form of ephedrine called *phenyl-propanolamine,* along with safe amounts of vitamins, benzocaine, and methyl cellulose. The stronger, more effective diuretics are sold by prescription only.

Most people get a better diuretic effect from cutting out salt and the heavily salted processed foods (see page 29). This is the healthy way to get rid of excess water. Susceptible people can lose too much potassium from taking too much of the mild diuretics. The labels on the drug mixtures of phenylpropanolamine, a mild diuretic, vitamins, benzocaine and methyl cellulose feature illusions to encourage you to think of yourself as thin. Often the large-print name on the label stresses appetite control or getting thin fast. An illustration of a thin model in a brief bathing suit is common to these preparations.

You will have to read the fine print on the label to find phenylpropanolamine, as well as the other ingredients. The catchy names of the mixtures in big print are to give you the *illusion* that the substance will slim you. If ephedrine really blocked appetite, no one would have a weight problem.

Ephedrine is the medicine in nose drops. It would take much more ephedrine than there is in the reducing mixtures to make the average adult *high.* And it's the potent property of getting people high that earned amphetamines their reputation. Amphetamines make you too high to want to eat. Or they might not—if you are one of the people who get hungrier after taking it.

Benzocaine, another ingredient of "safe" weight pills, is a local anesthetic. You will find it in skin creams for burns and insect bites.

I cannot believe that benzocaine can block appetite except by making susceptible people sick. Benzocaine is bad for allergic people. They should not use it on their skin. They should not take it internally.

Kelp, vitamin B_6, lecithin, and vinegar are foods, not drugs, that have been touted as aids in weight loss. They are harmless, but they do *not* melt fat away.

Prescription Medicine

The ideal weight-control drug would increase your basal metabolic rate and decrease your appetite.

These things would have to be done without harmful or unpleasant side effects.

Another ideal weight-control drug might block foods such as fat from being absorbed without blocking the foods your body needs for good nutrition.

There are no such drugs.

Back in the 1930s, there was a drug called *dinitrophenol* that raised basal-metabolic rate. People lost so much heat that they had slight fevers and always perspired while they were taking the drug. It became very popular because people could eat all they wanted and still lose weight.

A terrible thing happened after dinitrophenol was on the market for about six months. Many people came down with cataracts, suffered complete hair loss and liver damage. Dinitrophenol was promptly taken off the market.

Could this sort of thing happen again? It could.

What Do Amphetamines Do for Overweight?

Let's look into amphetamines in greater detail. Amphetamines—Benzedrine, Dexedrine, and others—don't increase basal metabolic rate the way dinitrophenol does—or did. Amphetamines don't actually stop hunger. They get you so jittery and shaky that you don't think about eating. Some people get headaches from being high and get sick to their stomach and vomit.

The chief action of amphetamines is on the brain and the nervous system. Susceptible people have had psychotic reactions from taking them. If amphetamines could safely suppress appetite, the overweight problem would have been solved long ago.

By now, many studies have been done on what amphetamines will and will not do. The United States Food and Drug Administration had a committee of experts review all the studies ("Anorectics Have Limited Use in Treatment of Obesity," FDA Drug Bulletin, Dec. 1972). Here is their opinion about all the amphetamines including the very latest ones:

> Most overweight people continue to eat after their appetite is satisfied whether they take an amphetamine or not. The average drop-out rate from

weight-loss programs is the same for people who don't take an amphetamine drug as for those that do.

The amphetamines listed below are the ones that were reviewed. Note that amphetamines that are not the exclusive property of a pharmaceutical company can be sold by any number of companies under different names. *Generic name* means the chemical or scientific name, and *proprietary name* means the brand name used by a drug company. In the long run, all the amphetamines have the same actions and the same side effects. The individual differences of the people who take the drugs have more bearing on effects of amphetamines than any differences between one amphetamine and another.

Generic Name	Propietary Name
Dextroamphetamine	Dexedrine, Biphetamine
Phenmetrazine	Preludin
Methamphetamine	Syndrox, Desoxyn
Benzphetamine	Didrex
Phendimetrazine	Plegine
Diethylpropion	Tenuate, Tepanil
Phentermine	Ionamine, Fastin
Chlorphenteramine	Pre-Sate
Fenfluramine	Pondimin
Clortermine	Voranil
Mazindol	Sanorex

The average weight loss is the same for people whether they take an amphetamine drug or not.
The risk of drug addiction, psychosis, mental depression, intense fears, hallucinations and insomnia are greater than any good the amphetamines have done for the overweight problem.

Recent, as yet inconclusive studies, suggest that birth defects may result from amphetamine use during pregnancy. The outcome of all the studies on amphetamines is that these are dangerous drugs. Widespread abuse of them has prompted strict government controls. Some experts believe amphetamines should be completely banned because there is widespread abuse in spite of government control and because experts find they are ineffective for weight loss over the long term. Even the few amphetamine-like drugs are considered by experts to be addicting and readily subject to abuse. Complete banning of amphetamines or the barring of doctors from prescribing all but a few amphetamine-like drugs for weight control is inevitable.

Most weight problems are chronic and recurring.

There is no place for short-term, dangerous drugs in a lifetime affair like weight loss and ideal-weight maintenance.

Do Hormones Have Anything to Do with Overweight?

Over 99 percent of overweight has nothing to do with hormones. Hormonal or glandular trouble is extremely rare compared to the number of people with weight problems.

Theories that hormonal imbalances cause overweight were popular before modern laboratory tests were developed. Now, we know for certain what the hormones do and don't do for overweight and weight control.

What Are the Facts About Thyroid Hormone?

A large number of thyroid pills have been prescribed for overweight people. The theory behind thyroid medication is that it increases basal metabolic rate.

It takes very large doses of thyroid to increase the basal metabolic rate. Small doses like one-quarter or one-half or even a whole grain of thyroid medication don't do much except interfere with the functioning of your own thyroid gland.

Any dose of thyroid medication that's big enough to increase your basal metabolic rate also increases your appetite. As soon as you stop taking the thyroid, your metabolic rate goes down, but it takes longer for your appetite to go down. You soon regain the weight you lost.

Another bad thing about weight loss from large doses of thyroid medication is that the weight you lose is mostly muscle and not fat.

But other things that are more dangerous to health happen from taking large doses of thyroid medication.

As many as 20 percent of people who take large enough doses of thyroid to increase their metabolic rates and cause weight loss get angina and hypertension.

People who take these large doses lose calcium from their bones.

There is cause for concern that the small doses of thyroid that many people take for years and years for weight problems may be one of the causes of osteoporosis in older Americans.

The known facts about thyroid hormone tell us that it shouldn't be taken for overweight. Thyroid hormone is only for people with proven thyroid disease.

The Facts About HCG

HCG stands for human chorionic gonadotropin.

It is made from concentrated urine from pregnant women.

The complete treatment of overweight with HCG consists of a 500-calorie diet, a little exercise, and injections of HCG.

Anyone will lose weight on a 500-calorie diet unless the person is completely motionless and confined to bed.

The claim for HCG is not that it *melts* fat—the 500-calorie diet does that. The claim is that HCG helps you stick to the 500-calorie diet without experiencing hunger and irritability.

The Food and Drug Administration says that HCG does *nothing* for weight control. This means that HCG has no effect on metabolism except at very high doses, where it causes side effects on sex glands and body changes similar to pregnancy changes. The FDA has ordered the manufacturers of HCG to put labels on the bottles that say HCG does nothing one way or another for weight loss.

Doctors who use HCG with a 500-calorie diet disagree.

How can we know whom to believe?

Let me first tell you something about the *placebo effect.*

The placebo effect means that if you want the medicine to work for you, it will.

It doesn't matter whether there's sterile water in the syringe or HCG. As long as you *want* results, it's *your will* and *your mind* working for you, not what's in the syringe.

It's my opinion that HCG works by way of the placebo effect.

The placebo effect of the hypodermic injection and the attention people get when receiving daily injections help them to stick to the 500-calorie diet. The 500-calorie diet causes weight loss.

But, in the long run, this is an expensive method.

The drug industry in North America is still searching for a safe, useful appetite depressant, but so far it has not come up with one.

SURGERY FOR FAT LOSS

Surgical removal of big fat pads has been done for years. And although it may sound simple, it has its share of complications. Fatty tissue does not heal well and is subject to wound infection after surgery. Wound infection is a possible complication when any surgery is done on a person who is more than twenty-five pounds overweight. Even necessary and lifesaving surgery is more hazardous as overweight increases.

Another operation to treat overweight is intestinal bypass, or jejuno-ileal shunt. The term comes from the anatomical names of the two portions of small intestine involved—jejunum and ileum. It is called a bypass or shunt because about eighteen inches of small intestine are not removed but bypassed by the flow of food. At a later time, the surgeon can reattach the eighteen inches of intestine to the mainstream of the intestine.

The purpose of this operation is to remove from the digestive process part of the food-absorbing surface of the small intestine, where most of our foods are absorbed. Note, however, that purified sugar is absorbed in the stomach and this absorption will take place in spite of the bypass.

The amount of weight that a person loses may be pretty high at first *because of the effects of surgery.* Just about everybody has a few weeks of upset after any major operation. There is appetite loss from the anesthesia and from simply subjecting the body to surgery. A major bowel operation has to heal before very much food can be eaten. During this time of recovery, everyone loses weight.

Very soon after an intestinal-bypass patient begins to eat the "normal" amount of food, the result is diarrhea. *Successful weight loss from the operation depends on diarrhea.*

The average bypass patient has been accustomed to eating between 5,000 and 7,000 calories or more a day. The only way for these calories not to get into the metabolism is for the food to flow out as diarrhea. The diarrhea can be so severe and cause such serious complications to health that another operation may be necessary to make the intestine intact again.

People who have gotten through a year with an intestinal bypass usually lose about half the weight they want to lose. At the end of a year, the weight loss tends to stop and weight levels off. This is because other parts of the small intestine gradually begin to absorb more food. Only about 45 percent of the men and women who have the operation get down to ideal weight. Thus the success of the intestinal bypass for weight loss is only fair.

Are there other complications besides severe diarrhea? Yes. The complications have been arthritis, liver trouble sometimes ending up as cirrhosis, kidney stones, malnutrition leading to tuberculosis, serious upsets of potassium and calcium levels in the body, and severe mental breakdown. People have died.

One-third or more of all those who have the operation have a serious medical or psychiatric complication. The death rate from medical complications after surgery at one of the best medical centers in the United States is at least 11 percent for this operation.

No one who weighs less than 300 pounds should consider taking the enormous risks involved.

The cost of the operation, including the intensive care that is necessary after surgery, often runs as high as $100,000.

The most meaningful lesson from the data on this operation is that the people who have gotten down to ideal weight are those who have changed their food and eating habits. They no longer eat 5,000 to 7,000 calories a day. They no longer eat mainly high-density foods.

FOOD, EATING, AND YOU

Lifetime Eating for Weight-Conscious People

8

Lifetime eating instead of "dieting" is common sense. You have conscious control over everything in your life connected with eating and food. Food and eating can be separated.

Lifetime eating puts the emphasis on new eating habits. It emphasizes the best kinds of foods for overweight people—and it emphasizes knowing why these foods are healthful for you.

Lifetime eating reverses the yo-yo process. Fast weight-loss diets urge you to count the hours till the diet is over and you can go back to your old food habits. With lifetime eating, you eat lean foods on ordinary days to feel full, get thin, and stay thin and healthy. Instead of picking a few days to go on a fad diet, you pick an occasional special day to enjoy a little of the high-calorie food that got you into trouble.

This is the way of eating that keeps many people thin and healthy.

Wade Holland, a restaurant reviewer based in the gourmet-restaurant city of San Francisco is thin and healthy. Wade and his family eat plain, lean, home-cooked meals on ordinary days. Their food choices are mostly plain vegetables and fruits, occasionally a little chicken. Slow eating and pleasant conversation are the rule. To review a restaurant meal, Wade has to eat as many as 2,500 calories at one sitting. But this happens only a few times a week. He doesn't get fat.

This way of eating is followed by many people whose business or professional obligations demand a certain number of high-calorie meals on occasion. They switch to very low density foods in between.

This is the way I eat. I eat low-density foods for health reasons as well. My Personal Genetic Health Score is very bad. But I also like to be thin. I feel better and have more energy. I love to eat; I have a big appetite. I would rather be full than eat any dessert except fruit. After a few years of putting my mind to it, I lost interest in ice cream, chocolate, cake—all desserts, in fact. I care about nothing except not being hungry and staying thin and healthy.

Lifetime weight control gives you a sense of self-confidence that your mind has power over your body and that something like rich food can't get the better of you.

How Do You Go About Lifetime Eating?

You have to make up your mind to accept the fact that you can't change the laws of nature. The basic law is that if you put more food energy into your body than you burn up, you'll gain weight.

You have to make up your mind that you'll get some healthful exercise to burn up more food energy.

Then *start changing your food habits by doing one thing at a time.*

Start by doing all the things to roll back your appetite that were suggested in Chapter 1.

Work at reorienting your taste buds. This will help decrease your appetite and make it easier for you to overcome nonhungry hunger. Stop eating the foods that urge you to eat more.

Every time you think about food, remind yourself that you are separating food and eating. Think of eating to live instead of living to eat.

Plan each day's food and menus ahead. Write them down and stick to them. Don't be pressured by the sight, smell, and habit of food. Don't go to the market when you're hungry.

You are better off buying natural foods and cooking from scratch—so you know for sure that you are eating only what you have decided to eat.

If you have to prepare food for growing children or others who have no weight problems, make a pact with yourself that you will not touch their food. You have to prepare your own *low-density* meals—and any other adults that you cook for will be better off eating the same food you eat.

If you have to nibble while preparing a meal, have raw-vegetable snacks right there on the counter so you can nibble safely.

Avoid leftovers by paying careful attention to portion sizes. Work at cooking only what will be eaten. Put all leftovers away for tomorrow, not for today. Put them away or throw them away. Don't be a human garbage can. If you are concerned with the starving children of the world, give some money to an organization that is working to help them.

Work out an eating schedule that will help you with your eating goals. If you can control your appetite better and feel better when you eat five or six small meals a day, divide your food that way. As long as you eat the right number of calories and the right foods, the number of meals you divide them into is up to you.

Be firm in your conviction not to eat or drink anything unless it is part of your nutrition and calorie needs.

Roll back your portion sizes. But remember, the more willing you are to change your food habits to low-density foods, the less you will have to cut portion sizes. Your genetic score should be an important factor in this decision. You can change your food tastes, but you can't change your genes.

If you can get yourself to acquire new eating habits and change your attitudes and tastes toward food and exercise, you can lose weight and maintain a new low weight as well as anyone else.

The longer you're overweight, the more firmly your self-image is fixed on fatness. It takes at least as long for your mind to get over that image as it takes your body to lose the weight. Make up your mind that once and for all you're going to keep it off and get a better image of yourself.

This takes time. It may take a year or two or more. How long it takes is completely up to you. What else can you do for yourself to solve your weight problem for life? Vow to yourself that you will not hide food in order to eat it secretly.

You can vow that you will be honest with yourself. You know by now that you can always find a doctor who will go along with your excuses and rationalizations. Most doctors do not want a confrontation. They figure that you're just a fatty with no will power and no self-assertiveness. The doctor rationalizes; "If I don't agree with these fat patients, they will only change doctors until they find a doctor who will go along with their excuses."

Do not get yourself into the trap of sweeping the truth under the rug just because you can get a doctor to go along with your rationalizations.

Start leveling with yourself now about how much you eat and what foods you eat.

Keep your food diary in a careful, truthful way.

Have a clear conscience so that you will be able to look at yourself in the mirror and see a thin body and an honest face.

Remember: When you're faced with any eating situation, *use your head.*

HOW TO MAINTAIN IDEAL WEIGHT FOR A LIFETIME

Anyone can maintain ideal weight for a lifetime.

It takes a new spirit of common sense, some basic food and eating knowledge, and a firm vow. You have to vow that you are certain that you can keep from gaining your weight back. You have to defy anyone who says you cannot stick to your vow.

The first thing to do is *make a contract with yourself* that you can and will keep your vow to maintain your ideal weight for a lifetime.

My Personal Ideal Weight Maintenance Contract

PASTE HERE

a photograph of yourself at
your ideal lifetime weight

My contract with myself:

I vow that I will not let myself down.

I vow that I will respect my body and my new, strong sense of inner
strength.

I vow that I can and will assert myself to eat to live instead of live to
eat.

Date _____   Signed _____

Witness _____

I WILL:

give up the foods that urge me to eat more.
eat slowly.
get over the "I cooked it, I have to eat it" complex.
write out a daily food plan and stick to it.
form good food and eating habits for my health and ideal weight.
buy only the foods on my shopping list.
make it my business to know the nutrition and food facts that will help
    me maintain my ideal weight and be healthy.
eat a good breakfast and a moderate lunch.

I WILL:

make dinner a beautiful experience on lean foods.
eat enough very low density foods at dinner so that I feel satisfied and can
    forget about food until the next morning.

eat pretty much the same foods at the same time every ordinary day to help me solve the problem of "What to eat?"*

eat only vegetables and a little low-density fruit for snacks.

do everything I can to shift my tastes and appetite down.

drink water with meals and more water in general.

always have low-density snacks and foods as well as break-the-rules foods when I invite my friends and relatives for special-occasion meals.

make healthful exercise part of my life.

choose low-density foods in restaurants.

leave food on my plate when I have to eat high-density foods at a restaurant.

plan ahead to do some extra exercise to make up for special-occasion eating.

set up a few realistic exceptions and stick to them.

remember that very small portions are the only way I can eat high-density foods.

I WILL:

use the smallest dish I can find for my favorite urging food and limit myself to one miniature helping a day.†

never refill my miniature dish.

Date	Signed
	Witness

I WILL NOT:

urge anyone to eat or let anyone urge me to eat or drink high-calorie foods, including alcohol.

feel guilty for declining someone else's offer of food.

go into the kitchen after dinner, except for "permissable snacks," see page 179

touch the refrigerator after dinner, except for "permissable snacks," see page 179

eat out of the refrigerator, cupboard, or off the kitchen counter.

eat in front of the TV.

eat any more fat than I absolutely have to.

eat foods with added sugars (corn syrup, honey, etc.) except in miniature, single helpings.

---

*Eating the same or similar foods every ordinary day helps you quit when you are full. This way of eating cuts out the Thanksgiving effect of foods that urge you to eat more.
†Think about shopping for a beautiful little dish that holds about a teaspoonful.

I WILL NOT:

eat any unnecessary foods because they tempt me, especially the foods composed mainly of fat.

eat fat just because it enhances a food.

feel that I am missing anything by not eating potato chips, nuts, pretzels, candy, crackers, fatty spreads, bacon, olives, malteds, and shakes.

eat the potato chips, French fries, or olives that are on my plate in restaurants or at parties.

do foolish things like starve myself and then eat 3,000 or 4,000 calories at one time. If I have to binge once in a while I will do it on raw vegetables.

eat at the movies unless I bring my own raw-vegetable snacks from home. I know that the butter on the buttered popcorn makes this snack high-density.

eat anything that is not on my daily food list.

eat food at any time without thinking about what it will do for my body and my health.

_____   _____
Date   Signed

                                _____
                                Witness

Look at the contract you have made with yourself every day and vow not to let any person or any event allow you to break it.

Nutrition Facts for Overweight People

9

"Nutrition" is concerned with what your body needs to get out of food for good health. It also involves what your body *does not* need from food for good health. You have to know some nutrition facts to plan the best way to eat for your health and weight.

Foods as they come from nature are mixtures of three big nutritional groups—protein, carbohydrate, and fat. Pure carbohydrate, fat, or protein foods have been processed in some way by some animal, but usually by humans. For example, honey is a pure carbohydrate processed by bees from parts of living plants. Butter is a pure fat and casein is a pure protein, both of which come from the processing of milk by humans. These single-component foods are relatively rare, but to explain basic nutrition, it helps to separate foods into three major groups as best as possible.

THE FACTS ABOUT PROTEIN

The muscle of your body is protein. Your skeletal muscles and your heart are the main places where your body has its protein. Your body also has protein in the walls (outer layers) of all the cells that make up your skin and internal organs. The walls of your fat cells, too, are protein.

How Much Protein Do You Need to Eat?

Everybody needs protein, but in differing amounts. Growing people need the most protein in their daily diet.

An unborn baby grows faster and more quickly than any other human and needs the most protein. Women who are pregnant need to eat between seventy and eighty grams of protein a day to provide for themselves and their baby. Nursing women need a little less—between sixty and seventy grams a day. Infants need about one gram of protein per pound of body weight.

Children from one to three years of age need about twenty grams of protein a day. From age three to ten they need thirty to thirty-five grams a day. Teenagers need between forty and sixty grams a day till they finish growing. Boys and girls who are shooting up at the rate of four or more inches a year need the higher amount. When teenagers finish growing, they need the average adult amount.

Sick people who have had surgery or are healing after an illness have individual, special needs for more than the average adult protein requirements.

The average adult who isn't pregnant, nursing, or sick needs no more than 30 to 40 grams of protein a day.

This estimate is based on several premises and assumes that we are talking about healthy adults who have been well nourished since infancy and early childhood.

For example, in the years before dialysis became available for patients with chronic kidney disease, special diets were essential for these people. Food protein increases the work of the kidneys because any excess nitrogen must be removed by the kidneys. Nitrogen is the chief element provided by protein that is not supplied by carbohydrate or fat. It was found that adults with chronic kidney failure who were stable—well and not ill with infection or a surgical condition—maintained their protein balance on as little as 20 grams a day of food protein.

An even more critical debate arose over growing children with serious kidney disease. Careful studies of protein balance showed that these children grew, albeit slowly, on as little protein as 15 grams a day.

In fact, an old but never disproved study at Stanford University (Slonaker, Stanford Univ. Publications) showed that rats given the highest amounts of protein when young to stimulate the fastest growth died sooner as adults if high protein was continued.

Large populations of the world have lived for centuries on nearly all plant sources of food. Meat was scarce and expensive. The key to protein nutrition among these people was and still is the mixing of plant proteins in order to eat a variety of amino acids, the building blocks of protein. Plant protein contains many, but not all, of the necessary amino acids. Traditional foods consisted of mixtures of grains and beans, for example, the rice and lentil mixture characteristic of India and the Mideast. Plant protein is so much less concentrated than animal protein and mixed with so much fiber, it is difficult to eat too much.

Modern scientific studies have shown that normal healthy adults can stay well and in protein balance with 30 to 35 grams a day of mixed plant protein. Cereals provided 62 percent of the protein in one study.

The high rates of occurrence of cholesterol diseases in the United States and Canada have prompted medical scientists to take the view that North Americans are eating too much protein. The excess is protein mixed with saturated fat. Studies of adults who eat no meat, only plant and a little fish protein, show that these people have lower blood cholesterols and other blood fats as well as lower body weights than the North American average.

Overweight people, unless they have some individual health condition, need even less protein than that. They have extra protein stored in their body in the form of enlarged skeletal muscles and fat-cell walls. Remember that one piece of meat, two inches by two inches and one-fourth-inch thick, contains seven grams of protein and five grams of fat (see page 202).

What Is the Best Way for Overweight People to Get Their Food Protein?

As every bit of fat you eat gives you a high-calorie load, weight-conscious people will want to choose protein mixed with as little fat as possible. The highest-density protein food—meaning the protein food with the most calories in the smallest volume—is nuts. This is because they are high in fat. Nuts have so much mixed-in fat compared to protein that they are usually listed as fats.

Here is a list of protein foods in order of their density, from highest to lowest:

Very High Density
Nuts
Peanut butter and peanuts

High Density
Meats and meat products, duck, goose
Chicken, turkey, game fowl
Cheese, most cheese products, and eggs
Milk except nonfat

Medium Density
Fish (fresh, water-packed canned fish, or canned fish with oil washed out)

Low Density
Fluid nonfat milk (it is common practice for 1 percent fat to be added to
    fluid nonfat milk. Powdered nonfat milk is truly nonfat.)
Vegetable protein (includes grains, beans, stems, roots and tubers)
Egg white

Is there a difference in the nutritional value of different protein foods? Yes. All proteins are composed of building blocks called amino acids. There are many amino acids, but eight of them are absolutely essential for human growth. All animal, fish, and fowl proteins contain all eight essential amino acids.

In order to get all the essential amino acids from vegetable protein, *you need to eat eat a mixture of vegetable-protein foods.* For example, corn protein has to be mixed with another vegetable protein such as beans, peas, or oats. *It is necessary to eat these combinations at the same meal.* Later in the day is not good enough. If you drink milk along with the vegetable protein, you will get all eight essential amino acids.

And as you lose weight, your body will be adding essential amino acids to your food protein from your broken-down fat cells.

In addition, all animal, fish, and fowl proteins, including egg white and milk, contain vitamin B_{12}. Vegetable proteins do not. Most adults need only a tiny amount of vitamin B_{12} two or three times a year.

Body changes such as those that occur during menstruation, pregnancy, and recovery from surgery or illness use up much more of the essential amino acids from food than when your body has no special jobs to do.

Does protein have any special qualities to help you lose weight? An old theory held that protein increases the amount of heat the body loses after a meal. But new research has completely refuted this.

Protein helps prevent hypoglycemia because it takes a long time to digest protein. The amino-acid building blocks of protein get into your metabolism very slowly. This slowness calls for small amounts of insulin to be made gradually by your pancreas. By preventing the hypoglycemia-hunger response, protein plays an important part in retraining your appetite and fullness feelings.

Are there protein foods that bring out genetic or nongenetic susceptibilities? Meat comes from nature with visible and invisible marbled fat. Animal fat, most of which is saturated, causes a lot of cholesterol production, especially in fat-sensitive people.

Too much fatty food causes overloaded metabolism in all people. But fat-sensitive people who have genetic weaknesses in their metabolism make too much triglyceride and cholesterol from food fat. So meats are *not* the best sources of protein for overweight people and they are particularly unwise choices for those with genetic fat-sensitivity diseases.

Nonfat milk is a *good* protein source for most overweight people. But some people cannot digest milk sugar because they don't have enough lactase in their intestinal tract. Lactase is the enzyme that digests milk sugar.

Yogurt is a form of milk that has the milk sugar already digested; the lactobacillus that changes milk to yogurt does the digestion for you. Nonfat

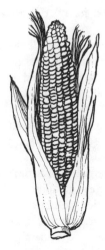

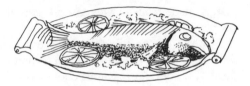

FISH
5½ oz., cooked

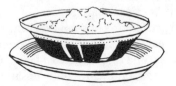

RICE
14 oz., dry *or*
OATMEAL
7 oz., dry

CORN
8¾ ears *or*
12 oz. of dry grits

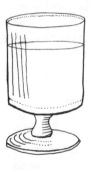

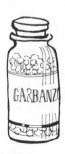

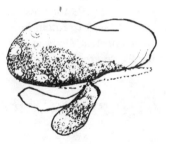

POTATO
9 medium, 3½" diam.

NONFAT MILK
27 oz.

GARBANZOS (CHICK PEAS)
4½ oz., dry

Each of these foods contains thirty grams of protein in the portion stated. (Thirty grams = one ounce.) A small amount of animal-origin protein, such as any nonfat milk product (like yogurt or cottage cheese), fish, very lean fowl, or egg white, adds essential amino acids. This supplement to plant protein gives you more complete protein because all essential amino acids are present. If you prefer to choose only plant-origin proteins, be sure to mix proteins from a variety of sources at each meal and also find a source of vitamin B12.

yogurt made from powdered milk is a good protein food for overweight people.

Fish is a fine protein food for overweight people because almost all the fat is right under the skin and can be removed. Shellfish contains almost no fat, but is high in exogenous cholesterol. Shellfish should be considered as a rare treat by overweight people with genetic susceptibilities—a food to break the rules with.

Chicken and turkey have very little marbled fat. Discard the skin and liver, which are fatty, get rid of all the fat you can, and use only the solid meaty portions that are lean.

Vegetable proteins are excellent sources for the overweight. They come from nature with less fat than animal and fowl proteins (except nuts and peanuts) and most vegetable fat is unsaturated. The exceptions are olive oil and coconut oil. Olive oil is unsaturated in nature, but it rapidly becomes saturated by human body metabolism. Coconut oil is saturated in nature.

Vegetable protein, as it comes from nature, also brings with it a great deal of bulk in the form of pulp (fiber). This bulk provides more volume than other protein foods (with the exception of the large water volume of nonfat milk) and helps you *feel full.*

See page 198 for a list of low-density protein foods of plant origin with the amount of protein in an average portion. On page 201, you will find a list of protein foods in portion sizes that contain seven grams of protein; foods are grouped in order of density from low to high.

THE FACTS ABOUT CARBOHYDRATE

Over half the people in the world stay thin on a high-carbohydrate diet. This is because they eat *low-density carbohydrate food* consisting of vegetables, fruits, and grains. Most carbohydrate foods are basically of plant origin. There is some carbohydrate in animal food (milk sugar, for example) but plants are the biggest source of carbohydrates.

Unless you mix considerable cooking fat or oil with these foods, you have to eat very large large quantities to build up much of a calorie load.

Nuts, seeds, avocado, chocolate, and olives are the big exceptions to the low density of natural carbohydrate foods. These plant foods contain large quantities of fat and should be avoided until you can stop eating after a miniature portion. Olive oil, safflower oil, sesame oil, soy oil, corn oil, peanut oil—all come from plants. When oil is the greatest part of a plant food, overweight people should avoid that food.

Sunflower seeds also contain contain large quantities of oil. Overweight people should never eat shelled sunflower seeds. If you have to shell them yourself, it takes so long you won't eat very many.

Corn and soybeans differ from other oily seeds in that in nature their oils are mixed with much more pulp. If you want to eat corn and soybeans, it is best not to add fat or oil.

Can You Lose Weight on High-Carbohydrate Diets?

It is possible for a person to plan a lifetime diet of all plant foods that will have the proper amount of protein, essential amino acids, calcium and other minerals, and all vitamins except B_{12}. Most North Americans who eat this way take some dairy products once or twice a week, some fish once a week, and some eggs once or twice a month. They add these foods for variety, for additional protein, and to get Vitamin B_{12}.

The purpose of these people is not necessarily to lose weight. However, studies show that these people all lose weight for the first two years. The important fact for overweight people is that North Americans who switch to plain vegetarian diets do lose weight and report that they are full, satisfied, and not hungry.

These people who eat high-carbohydrate, low-density foods gradually lose the extra fat padding that we have come to take for granted. Their blood cholesterol is lower than average, because they eat very little fat and they stay thin.

Plant Foods

In addition to helping weight loss and lowering cholesterol, plant foods make your digestive tract work hard because the foods have their basic calorie-giving chemicals locked in between layers of pulp.

Your teeth have to do lots of chewing, your digestive juices have to work hard, and your stomach and intestines have to put out their best effort to get the nutrients out of the pulp. The leftover fiber helps your intestines sweep away waste products and prevents constipation. And fiber from *mixtures of plant food* doesn't concentrate phytic acid as straight bran does (see page 111.)

Two grams a day is the amount of fiber you need. This is supplied by *any one* of the following foods:

      Small portion of whole-wheat cereal (3½ ounces)
      3 average-sized carrots
      2 average-sized turnips
      1 medium-sized apple
      1 artichoke
      Small portion of cooked or raw peas (3½ ounces)

There is a complete list of fiber-containing foods on page 203.

Other factors than pulp keep the calorie density of vegetables low. Vegetables store energy in the form of starch. Humans do not digest all of the starch and sugar calories out of vegetables, especially raw vegetables.

Animals, called ruminants, which get all their calories and nourishment from plant food, can digest every bit of the starch and protein from plant food. These animals have an extra stomach chamber, a *rumen,* that digests the pulp part of leaves, grasses, and grains during the night while the animal sleeps.

Humans do not have this extra stomach chamber. We initiate the breaking-down process by cooking. When you eat vegetables raw—carrots, peas, turnips, beets and onions, for example—you get fewer calories than when you eat them cooked. You can't digest out all the calories from raw vegetables. When you eat foods in their natural forms, you get the benefit of all the pulp as well as all of the minerals in the skins—and fewer calories.

Eating natural foods means that no edible portion has been removed, that no taste enhancers (sweeteners, fats, salt, or spices) have been added. Natural foods are very nutritious as well as filling.

Do not confuse natural food and organic food. The term *organic* refers only to the kind of fertilizer used to grow a crop and the kind of insecticides used.

What About Processed Carbohydrates?

Wheat. When wheat is processed, the first step is to grind it up. Coarsely ground wheat is eaten as cereal. Finely ground wheat is used for flour. If no parts are removed, it is whole-wheat flour.

Often, however, the bran part of wheat is taken off and sold separately. The bran, like the wall of the human cell, contains a lot of protein. But it also contains a lot of iron-blocking phytic acid. The germ part of the wheat is also taken off and sold separately. The germ, like the nucleus of the human cell, contains protein. Both the bran and germ contain trace minerals and vitamins.

The remaining white flour is nearly pure starch. Though the vitamins are often replaced and the product sold as "enriched" flour, you still are not getting the benefit of trace minerals.

Flour, like all starch, contains only four calories to the gram. A teaspoon is four grams—sixteen calories. But starch such as flour is almost always mixed with fat or sugar or both.

With flour, as with any purified starch or sugar, you get a smaller volume of food to eat than if you ate the grain in its natural form. If you eat whole wheat, you also get protein to fill your protein need. Bread made from whole wheat is a good food if you can eat it without fat and sugar.

Rice. The rice story is a little different.

The natural wall covering rice is also bran. Rice bran has more protein than wheat bran. But centuries ago, it became fashionable to eat polished rice. As the fad for polished rice spread, so did vitamin-B deficiencies. The vitamin-B content in rice is high, but the vitamin B is in the covering. Today, rice is lightly polished and often fortified with vitamins. Rice and other whole-grain foods are good carbohydrate foods for overweight people. Brown rice is the same as other rice in protein content. It is significantly higher in phosphorus content. With rice, you get a large volume of food to eat in relation to the number of calories.

The best way to eat grains is with other food, such as beans and legumes, that enhance the flavor and add essential amino acids without adding many calories.

Processed Sugar. There are also unnatural carbohydrates—the processed sugars. When your body digests the starch and sugar out of foods in their natural form, your metabolism gets the sugar out of the pulp in a slow, gradual way. When your body gets sugar that has already been processed, your metabolism is hit all at once by a rapid-fire load of sugar.

Raw sugar or incompletely processed sugar is no different in its effect on your body than pure white refined sugar. Raw sugar is simply not bleached; it's still sugar without any pulp.

When you ingest a lot of processed sugar at one time, your pancreas produces a large quantity of insulin. Down goes your blood sugar. You soon feel hungry again or headachy or sleepy or have some other symptom special to your body. All forms of sugar can cause the hypoglycemic response.

In a sense, sugar is *addictive* because of the hypoglycemic response it can cause. You are dependent on getting more sugar in order to feel better.

The commonest raw materials for table sugar are sugar cane and sugar beets. An inexpensive and not very difficult process extracts the sugars from the plants and purifies it into *sucrose.*

Cane or beet, the chemistry is the same. Sucrose is a two-part sugar. The parts are *fructose* and *glucose.*

Glucose is normal body sugar. We all need glucose. But fructose is a highly suspect sugar. The evidence is growing that many people have a genetic weakness for making blood fat from overloads of fructose.

Humans have been getting fructose in fruits for millions of years. But the fructose in natural fruit is mixed with pulp. The amount of fructose you actually get out of a piece of fruit is small. It has to be digested out of the pulp compartments in a slow and gradual process. After it is digested out of the pulp, it is slowly and gradually absorbed down the whole length of the intestinal tract, not taken directly into the bloodstream from the stomach.

When fructose is absorbed slowly and gradually, your sugar metabolism has a chance to change fructose to glucose. But big doses of purified fructose overload the sugar metabolism. People with genetic sugar weakness and genetic triglyceride weakness are especially likely to be victims of overloaded sugar metabolism.

Glucose itself in too large quantities coming on too rapidly also causes the hypoglycemic response the same way sucrose does. Both glucose and fructose are quickly absorbed. The glucose is added to the already sufficient amount of glucose in the body. The fructose part overloads sugar and fat metabolism.

The amount of pure fructose is increasing in commercially prepared foods.

Fructose by itself is sweeter than glucose by itself or sucrose. A new economical process to change corn syrup to *all* fructose was perfected in 1974. Corn syrup is now purified fructose.

Commercial food processors claim that less fructose will sweeten more food and that the end result will be fewer calories. *Those fewer calories are not of any consequence to people with weight problems.* The possible health hazards from purified fructose are under intensive scientific study by prestigious scientists. In the meantime, it is common sense for overweight people to avoid processed foods sweetened with corn syrup.

Sucrose does more than sweeten foods. It enhances food in a number of ways. It preserves food, enhances taste, and provides bulk, gloss, texture, and aromas that chemists have not been able to equal with glucose or artificial sweeteners. But in addition to causing the hypoglycemic response, sucrose contributes greatly to the overloaded metabolism, overweight, and diabetes, and causes dental caries.

Brown sugar is unbleached sucrose. Molasses and sorghum come from the bottom of the barrel of the sucrose-refining process. Honey is another form of sugar, processed by bees in nature.

Honey, brown sugar, molasses, and sorghum contain minerals that refined sugar lacks. However, these types of sugar have the same basic components as sucrose. They are all composed of fructose and glucose. They are all rapidly absorbed and can cause the hypoglycemic response.

Are there any substitutes for sucrose and fructose? Glucose, the normal body sugar, has never been popular as a sweetener because it is not as sweet as sucrose. You will find glucose in some diet foods, under the name of *sorbitol.* Glucose or glucose under another name is still four calories per gram. Pure glucose still has the disadvantage of being absorbed all at once, causing the hypoglycemic response.

There is no question that our bodies need glucose. But we need only small amounts of it. Our bodies function best if we have to work for every bit of glucose by using the efforts of our digestive tract to get the sugar out of its natural pulp coverings and compartments.

Common sense, prevention of cavities, and health sense, especially for all with a genetic weakness for disease from overloaded metabolism, call for a personal ban on sugar. Yet it is difficult to put a personal ban on sugar. You will find suggestions for how to go about doing it on pages 136–137 and 158.

THE FACTS ABOUT FAT

Fat and oil are the same when it comes to calories. Each supplies nine calories per gram, twice as many as carbohydrates and proteins.

The difference is that fat is solid and oil is liquid at room temperature. In other words, fat is solid oil. Oil is liquid because it is less "saturated" in its internal chemistry than fat.

Cholesterol belongs to the fat group of substances and is made in the bodies of all animals.

How Much Fat Do We Need in Our Diet?

Babies and small children need fat in their diet for the important growth job of finishing the coverings of nerves and certain parts of the brain. Growing children don't need much fat. Overweight adults and teenagers need as little fat in their diet as they can possibly get away with.

The human body was programmed millions of years ago to get along on sparse amounts of plant food but to be able to store energy from rare feasts of meat. Now that we have an abundance of food, shelter, and clothing, we don't need to store fat and we don't need a protective layer of fat to keep us warm.

The average North American eats 20 to 30 percent or more calories in the form of fat daily. This fat consumption represents food tastes, habits, and customs. It has nothing to do with good nutrition.

There is enough fat in natural seeds and grains to take care of all the nutritional needs of overweight people.

If you eat a small amount of fish or fowl on occasion, you will be getting more than enough fat.

If your Personal Genetic Health Score is positive, you are better off without any saturated fat in your food. Saturated fat is very likely to be made into endogenous cholesterol by your metabolism. Cut out saturated fat except for special-occasion foods.

Polyunsaturated Fat

If you eat polyunsaturated fat in exchange for all the saturated fat you have been eating, your cholesterol level will come down, provided you do these things:

- Stop overloading your metabolism. In other words, lose weight.
- Cut way back on all foods that contain exogenous cholesterol.
- Remember that polyunsaturated fat still contains nine calories per gram.
- Remember that one-fourth teaspoon is one gram.

It's very easy to get too many calories if you're eating more than a tiny amount of fat.

When you are gaining weight, every food, including polyunsaturated fat, can provide the building blocks for cholesterol made by your body.

Even a negative Personal Genetic Health Score is not a guarantee against cholesterol diseases if you overload your metabolism. Overweight people shouldn't look for ways to add polyunsaturated fat to their food; they should seek ways to reduce the amount of all fats and oils they eat.

Remember that the best way to lower your blood cholesterol is to lose weight.

As all animal-origin foods—milk, meat, eggs, fish, shellfish, and fowl—have *some* cholesterol in them, you will want to know more about these foods. The more cholesterol your body makes, the less you should eat from food sources. There is a list of foods high in exogenous cholesterol on page 214. On page 215, you will find a list of fatty foods grouped according to how much polyunsaturated compared to saturated fat they contain.

Remember that all fat foods have a big calorie impact. When you choose to eat any of them, the more unsaturated ones are better. But the lowest amount of fat you can get down to is best of all. (There is a list of natural foods that are high in fat on page 216.)

THE FACTS ABOUT VITAMINS

People who are growing or whose bodies are changing fairly rapidly need extra vitamins. Overweight people who are on fad diets or very restricted diets need extra vitamins because their bodies are changing very rapidly.

Otherwise, we need only small amounts.

Each vitamin does a small but specific job in the body. If you choose a lifetime diet that is high in fruits, grains, and vegetables, you don't have to take extra vitamins unless you decide to eat no animal-origin food. Then you have to take in a small amount of vitamin B_{12}. Remember that B_{12} is found in milk, yogurt, and all milk products. If you eat fish, seafood, or some kind of fowl once in a while, you will get all the vitamin B_{12} you need. Unless, of course, you have a special problem that requires increased vitamin B_{12}.

If you are overweight from drinking too much alcohol or soft drinks, or from eating too many sweets or too much highly processed food, you may not be getting enough vitamins.

On pages 210–213, you will find lists of foods high in vitamins A, the B complex, C, D, E, and K.

THE FACTS ABOUT MINERALS

If you are overweight because you eat or drink too many sweets, too much processed food, soft drinks, and alcohol, you can also be courting a mineral deficiency. These foods are short of iron and calcium. They are also short of trace minerals—minerals needed by the body in minute quantities. These include copper, selenium, zinc, magnesium, and sulfur.

Trace amounts of copper and selenium have a place in that all-important cholesterol metabolism and help to keep blood cholesterol down. The only way to get these trace minerals is to eat a wide selection of natural foods and to eat vegetables with the skin on (after scrubbing it well) instead of peeling the vegetables and throwing the skin away. The root vegetables, potatoes, carrots, beets, turnips, parsnips, and rutabagas can be scrubbed instead of peeled.

Carbonated drinks are very high in phosphorus, which tends to pull calcium out of the bones. Unless you eat foods containing calcium, you should avoid a high-phosphorus diet.

Did you know that there is calcium and magnesium in the skin of potatoes? When you eat potatoes with the skins removed, you get only the phosphorus and not the calcium and magnesium.

In nature, it is normal to find calcium, magnesium, and phosphorus in balance. You find this balance in milk and other foods containing calcium and phosphorus. For good nutrition, it's smart to eat foods with the minerals in natural balance.

Most root vegetables, like potatoes, have calcium in their skins. If you throw away significant parts of the these foods, you will be getting rid of minerals such as calcium, zinc, copper, selenium, and magnesium.

Taking calcium or other minerals in the form of tablets is hazardous. It's very easy to take too much. Kidney stones are caused by taking too much calcium. This is especially true in people who have a genetic susceptibility to kidney stones and other calcium diseases.

There are lists of high-calcium foods and of high-phosphorus foods on page 208.

Note that milk contains calcium and phosphorus but no iron.

There is a list of foods high in iron on page 209.

Now it's your move.

There are compelling reasons for changing to low-density, lean eating:

> To unload your metabolism
> To lose weight
> To learn lifetime food and eating habits while you unload your metabolism and lose weight
> To roll back your tastes and re-educate your taste buds to dislike greasy tastes and sensations in your mouth and to dislike too much sweet and salt
> To learn how to turn your back on foods that urge you to eat more
> To learn how to transfer to very low density snacks when you have to nibble

Anyone can lose weight. You don't have to go hungry.

You *do* have to learn to eat to live instead of living to eat.

Rich foods that urge you to eat more are so abundant, you have to work toward having complete conscious control over everything connected with food and eating. Every decision about, "What should I eat?" brings up your health as well as your body size and shape.

If your Genetic Health Score is six or more on each side of your family, start now, the younger the better, to learn the low-density way to eat to live. If you have few or no genetic worries about health from overweight, you have to decide whether you prefer small portions of high-density food or large portions of low-density food.

The more high-density food you eat, the more carefully you have to watch your calorie count. Face up to it realistically: One cheeseburger with French fries, one ice-cream soda, and one piece of pie add up to the total daily calories needed by the average North American woman. The average man can add one glazed donut.

This is not very much food. But it's loaded with calories.

The more weight you have to lose and the larger your appetite, the easier it is to succeed on low-density food. You can eat large amounts while getting a small calorie impact.

It's your move.

You have to take the responsibility for knowing what you're doing and why, or you will never succeed.

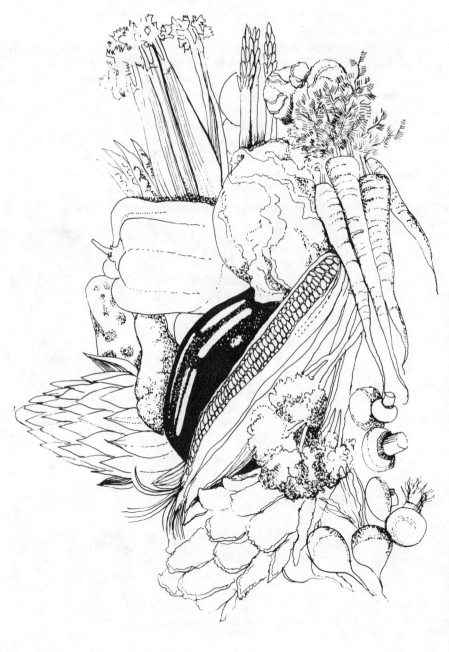

Very low density food. See Lists 8, 9, and 11 on pages 198, 201, and 205 for classifications of foods according to density.

Lifetime Foods for Weight-Conscious People 10

Once you've made up your mind to eat only for your body's needs, your battle is nearly won. Your goal is gradually to get yourself happy, full, and thin with the lowest-density foods that will satisfy your body's needs.

You must plan your food strategy so you will not be hungry. It can take a long time to change your food habits. But if you have trouble with nonhungry hunger, it's easier to change your food habits than your eating habits.

How Do You Change Your Food Habits?

First, stop eating all high-density favorite foods.

Make up your mind that your favorite food or foods are taboo. Tell yourself: "I can't eat that." Tell your friends or hostess: "I'm not allowed to eat that."

Stop enhancing fruit, cereal, and bread with sweeteners. Stop putting sugar, honey, or molasses on your foods.

Switch to low-density, safe foods for the times you feel you have to nibble.

Make a contract with yourself that for three months you won't eat any of your favorite foods that urge you to eat more. Mark the date on the calendar. At the end of three months, ask yourself if you feel you missed anything. Sign up for another three months.

Write an essay for yourself on what it meant to you to give up the foods that urged you to eat more. Be sure to write about whether you missed them and for how long. Write about how long—how many weeks or months—it took before being full was more important to you than what you ate.

Can You Change Your Drinking Habits?

Water is the best low-calorie drink you can find. Remember that all soda —diet or regular—contains phosphorus, which removes calcium from bones. Sweetened drinks add too many calories to be worth the pleasure they might bring. Learn the joy of drinking plain water.

Drinking water with your meals helps you eat more slowly and helps fill you up with less food. It helps break up the flow of solid food into the intestines and counteracts constipation. At mealtime, put a glass of water at each place on the table.

If you can't stand plain water, add some safe, noncaloric flavoring. Tea or coffee, of course—or just a few drops of peppermint flavoring. Water can be flavored by boiling it with mint leaves, orange peel, lemon peel, cloves, cinnamon, or herbs. Cap it tightly and store it in the refrigerator. It's also possible to break the sweet-drink habit by adding spices to tea.

Nonfat milk helps fulfill your protein needs while supplying water for the body. Noncaloric flavorings like coffee, tea, or vanilla help some people enjoy nonfat milk.

Fruit juices contain natural fruit sugar, which has the same number of calories as refined sugar. Fruit juice does not have the advantages of making your digestive processes work and giving you the fullness feeling of the whole fruit. You are better off eating a whole orange or grapefruit. If you want to drink juices instead of water, choose those with the lowest amount of fruit sugar—tomato and grapefruit juice.

Alcoholic beverages increase appetite in three ways: by irritating the stomach lining and increasing the feeling of hunger; by relaxing tension; by causing the hypoglycemic response. Hypoglycemia is such a significant appetite increaser, you will want to avoid it every way you can. If you have to drink to relax, count the calories. The higher the proof, the higher the alcohol content and the more calories you get. See page 192 for a formula you can use to figure the number of calories in drinks.

Try to step down a notch or two in the calorie content of alcoholic beverages. Sweetened alcoholic drinks have to be given up. If you can't stand alcoholic beverages unless they're sweet, you are lucky. Quit.

If you have to have your drink, go down from the highballs to small amounts of wine or beer. Make a firm contract with yourself to limit your alcohol intake to four ounces or less of dry wine or twelve ounces or less of beer in twenty-four hours. If you can't stick to that contract, you may have a drinking problem in addition to a weight problem.

How Do You Decide How Many Calories to Eat?

The average woman will lose weight eating 1,200 calories a day. In order to maintain a new low weight, she will not be able to eat more than 1,400 to 1,600 calories a day.

The average man will lose weight on 1,500 calories a day. In order to maintain a new low weight, he will not be able to eat more than 1,800 to 2,000 calories a day.

An exercise program will help you feel better, sleep better, stay in better condition and allow you to eat a little more food.

Learn to estimate the calories in mixtures of food. The majority of calorie counts on labels of prepared and processed food are based on estimates—educated guesses based on what foods went into the mixture.

The Break the Rules Calorie Counter on page 222 will help you learn calorie estimates. For example, all meat casseroles are alike enough for you to judge one against another for practical calorie counting.

How Do You Decide What Foods to Eat?

First, you must decide what foods not to eat.

Foods that are high in salt don't make sense for overweight people. Stop salting your food at the table.

Highly salted foods interfere with the sodium-potassium balance and add to the problems of water retention. If you have hypertension, you have more than one reason to cut out added salt.

You will find a list of natural foods and the amount of salt they contain on page 193. A list of processed and prepared foods and the amount of salt they each contain appears on page 195. You will see that the foods in the second list contain large amounts of salt. This is one reason that processed and prepared foods should be avoided. Eating salt is a habit that grows on you and urges you to eat more and more.

Potassium is the natural protector of the body against salt. See page 197 for a list of foods that are high in potassium.

Foods that contain a lot of fat don't make sense for overweight people. Your body has more fat than it needs. Eat no more fat than you have to.

Memorize the list of highest density foods composed mostly of fat (see page 207). Make a contract with yourself not to eat any of these foods for three months. If any of them is your favorite urging food, it has to be stopped anyway.

Powdered cream substitutes are saturated fat. If you must have a lightener for your tea or coffee, switch to a safe substitute such as powdered nonfat milk.

Cut down on fats and oils as much as possible. The closer you can get to cutting fat and oil out of your foods, the easier weight maintenance will be for you. The natural oils in grains and fresh vegetables are all your body needs.

Enhancing foods with fat and oil is a habit just like oversalting and feeding the sweet tooth. There is nothing wrong with bread and potatoes, for example, except the fat we are in the habit of enhancing them with.

Teach your taste buds to dislike the taste and feel of fat. Think of fat as greasy and unhealthful. Learn to cook and eat without fat. Practical suggestions for cooking without fat appear in Chapter 11. When you do use fat, be sure it's unsaturated. See page 215 for practical information about the polyunsaturated-fat content of fat foods.

Satisfy your craving for sweets with fruit. If sweets are your downfall, you have to cut them out. You have to eat fruit for dessert. Commercial gelatin desserts are high in refined sugar, for example, and many commercial products are sweetened with purified fructose.

A sweet tooth is one of the hardest taste habits to turn off. Rise above it. Assert yourself. You have to substitute fruit without added sugar or artificial sweetener or your weight loss and health goals are pipe dreams.

At this point, if you still want to know how you can eat all the candy, cake, pie, donuts, crusts, ice cream, whipped cream, meats, bacon, mayonnaise you want without getting fat, the answer is *you can't.*

There is one common-sense alternative. Teach yourself to want these foods only on special occasions. That's the only way you can fit them into the realities of body energy consumption and output.

First, you need to teach your taste buds to enjoy the foods that are best for your body. Then you will be the proud owner of a set of lasting rules. When you know the rules, you can break them once in a while at *your* will. To help you break the rules intelligently, you will find the Break the Rules Calorie Counter on page 222.

What Foods Can You Eat?

Protein is something everyone needs (see page 139). It is possible to get your protein needs from vegetable foods alone. Vegetable protein, nonfat milk, and egg white are the lowest-density protein foods. Except for the small amount of exogenous cholesterol in nonfat milk, there is no exogenous cholesterol in low-density protein foods. Low-density protein sources give you the largest amount of food to eat with the lowest calorie intake.

Plan your food for the day around your protein need. Remember to eat a mixture of vegetable protein foods to get all the essential amino acids. You can get complete protein by mixing wheat, oats, and corn, rice, millet, and any of the beans and other legumes. If you eat a nonfat milk product, you get complete protein and vitamin B_{12}, which is absent in vegetable foods. If you add some fish to your diet, you needn't use nonfat milk products unless you want to. If you add some egg white to your menu, you add vitamin B_{12} and essential amino acids.

It makes sense to look into the low-density proteins eaten by so many people of other parts of the world. The nutrition secret of the Orient is to mix grains and legumes—rice is mixed with lentils, a high-protein legume, or with a variety of soybean products. Chick peas (also called garbanzos or ceci) are high in protein and much of the population of the Middle East eats them for breakfast.

You will find a list of the many vegetable foods that are high in protein on page 198. A small number of fruits contain a fair amount of protein. Menu suggestions and recipes for low-density protein food appear in Chapter 12.

Remember that the lower the density of your protein food, the more you get to eat and the less likely you are to lose your courage because of hunger.

Compare the volume of food you get to eat when you eat low, medium, high, and very high density protein foods by looking at the list on page 201. Each food is listed with the portion that supplies you with seven grams of protein. One slice of bologna, one-eighth inch thick, for example, supplies you with seven grams of protein and also five grams of fat.

When you go on a fad or crash diet, you need to take vitamins. When you follow a low-density diet for life, you get all the vitamins you need: A and D, the different B vitamins, vitamins C and K, and all whole grains and seeds are high in vitamin E.

Low-density eating also provides all the fiber you need for a daily intake of two grams. Carrots and turnips have some of the most healthful of all food fiber. Or you may prefer celery, green pepper, cucumber, bean sprouts, raw cauliflower, or zucchini. For a complete list of high-fiber food, see page 203.

When you go food shopping, have your grocery list in hand. Take only enough money to buy the things on your list. Build your daily food plan around the amount of protein you need and start thinking about getting your protein in the lowest-density forms possible. Don't buy anything not on your list unless it's a special on fresh vegetables or fruits in season.

11

Cooking Facts for Overweight People

There are many reasons why overweight people should prepare their own foods from scratch. The first is to get all the important minerals, including trace minerals, that are lost in commercially prepared foods. Overweight people are notoriously malnourished, especially in iron, calcium, and trace minerals. The next is to help cut the salt habit. Another is to decrease the amounts of fat and sugar in foods. And working with natural ingredients to build tasty dishes will help you learn more about calories and portion sizes.

Suggestions for Food Preparation

There are a number of ways to cook without using fat. If you stop using fat as a food enhancer, it has only one use left—to prevent sticking. If you must use something to prevent sticking, use spray-on nonstick vegetable oil. By spraying it on, you get an almost negligible amount of fat.

Alternative cooking methods include just about any of the usual ways, but always with the goal of using the least amount of fat.

Have you ever tried *barbecued vegetables?* One weekend, I was invited to give a talk on nutrition to a group of young men and women in training to do voluntary paramedical work in Third World countries. The Friday evening icebreaker was a barbecue dinner with a community salad bowl and bring-your-own steak. I brought two huge carrots for myself and put them over the hot coals. I should have brought more. By the time everyone had sampled the tasty morsels, I had hardly a bite for myself. I happen to like carrots, but there is no vegetable that does not become a gourmet delight when barbecued. Whether you use a barbecue or a hibachi or some other kind of cooking-over-hot-coals arrangement, fish as well as vegetables take on a summer-gala flavor when cooked this way.

Poaching is a fat-free cooking method particularly good for fish. If you think that fish has to be laden with oil and breading, you will be pleased to know about poaching. All the method requires is a two-quart pot half-filled with water. You can add some cooking wine, bay leaf, parsley, pepper corns, coriander, sesame seeds, and lemon peel if you wish, and bring the water to a boil. The average slice of fish (from six to nine ounces) takes about ten minutes to cook. Your fish is done when it can be flaked with a fork.

Steaming is a very fast method for cooking fruits, vegetables, and grains. The commonest ways to steam-cook are to place a colander or a steamer unit in a pot and bring the water to a boil. The water level should be about one-half inch below the steamer so that the food never sits in water. When the water is boiling, add the vegetables, cover the pot, and lower the flame. When vegetables are cut in similar-size pieces, they will cook at the same rate. The average cooking time for three-fourths-inch to one-inch pieces is four to seven minutes.

Baking creates taste sensations different from those produced by any of the other cooking methods. Squashes, yams, potatoes, tomatoes, and onions are very tasty sprinkled with chopped parsley, chives, or other herbs of your choice. Wrap them in aluminum foil and bake till the taste and consistency suit you.

Sautéing is a method of pan-frying in which food is left on the fire for the shortest possible time. It is possible to sauté vegetables until they are just beginning to soften, without using oil. Simply add a few teaspoons of water or wine each time your vegetables begin to stick. Try browning diced onions under the broiler and then sautéing them for a few minutes with beans or legumes that have already been cooked. Spinach and mushrooms are delightful sautéed. Take one bunch of well-washed spinach, including the stems, and shred it. Dice in a few small pieces of ginger root and a clove of garlic. Add one teaspoon of soy sauce and sauté the mixture for three or four minutes. When you want to break the rules, a fourth of a teaspoon of sesame seed oil (available where Oriental foods are sold) brings out an exotic flavor you never knew spinach had. Mushrooms are very tasty when sautéed lightly with a little browned onion. Try adding some peas, either fresh or frozen to this mushroom mixture. Mushrooms are high in protein and one of the lowest-density foods you can find. Lettuce is a treat sautéed with a little soy sauce.

Broiling is another good way to get flavor differences out of vegetables. Be sure to cut root vegetables into very thin slices and turn or mix your vegetables every few minutes so they do not burn. Baking and broiling will bring tastiness out of celery that has amazed many men and women who formerly believed vegetables were only for rabbits.

Microwave cooking is another suitable method for low-density cooking. It is also useful for weight-conscious people who hate to cook; you can cook and eat in the same food containers. The rapid cooking of the microwave equals the speed of the fastest cooking methods. Both fruits and vegetables can be cooked with little or no water and no fat or oil.

Pressure cooking is another way to cook grains, beans, and legumes. You have to be sure you add enough water and never open the lid till the pressure has had a chance to normalize.

A Chinese *wok* is an ideal way to steam or sauté vegetables. You need a gas stove to use a wok, but you don't need to use oil, only water, stir continuously to make sure your vegetables do not burn.

The choices of cooking methods are so many that if you enjoy cooking, you can experiment for years.

Many people avoid cooking *dried beans and legumes* because they believe these foods have to be presoaked. Experience has shown that presoaking is not necessary. The faster-cooking dried beans and lentils cook on the stove top in about forty minutes and in about twenty minutes in a microwave oven. Soybeans take the longest to cook of all these foods and require the most water.

You can cook *mixtures of grains* either by steaming them or placing them in a microwave oven. Remember that mixtures of grains help you to get complete protein because they supplement each other's essential amino acids. Whole wheat, either cracked or unground, cooks nicely when mixed with rice, barley, or millet. You can mix legumes with grains and cook them all together if you wish.

Hard root vegetables such as beets, rutabaga, potatoes and yams, and parsnips can be steamed, baked, broiled, sautéed, or cooked in a microwave oven. For broiling and sautéing, cut them into thin pieces. For the other methods, larger pieces are suitable. *Don't peel your root vegetables.* Get a vegetable scrub brush and scrub the outsides. Keep the important minerals and trace minerals in the skins for your nutrition.

You may want to barely soften hard root vegetables; then chill them, and cut them into sticks and shapes for hors d'oeuvres and snacks. Steaming or microwave-cooking them for four or five minutes will do the job.

Fresh *corn on the cob* is one of summer's delights. You can cook it in a steamer in three or four minutes. You can cook corn inside of a paper bag in a microwave oven. You can cut it off the cob and add it to salads and cooked vegetable mixtures. Corn contains protein, three and one-half grams in one medium ear; that is one-sixth of the average daily protein requirement for an overweight adult. It also contains some quantity of all the minerals, trace minerals, and vitamins. Teach yourself to eat corn without any flavor enhancers. You will find that fresh, lightly cooked corn has a flavor all its own waiting to be discovered.

Crisp vegetables such as bean sprouts (any type of bean can be sprouted), onions, celery, green pepper, all types of lettuce, mushrooms, summer squash, zucchini squash, thin slices of root vegetables, spinach, and tiny corn cobs can all be steamed together or cooked together in a microwave oven. You can add peas, pea pods, string beans, and fresh lima beans. In fact, you can put together any mixture of vegetables that the season permits. Don't overcook. When you can smell the vegetable, it's done.

Summer fruits such as early varieties of nectarines and peaches taste sweeter and you will find it easier to separate pulp from seed if you cook them very briefly. Two minutes of steaming or microwave cooking are enough. Brief cooking will also afford you instant ripening of not-quite-ripe pears, peaches, plums, and nectarines.

You can barely soften—cook *al dente*—summer fruits with no added sugar and *freeze* them for use all through the fall, winter, and spring. You can do the same with any vegetable. Steaming or microwave cooking preserves the vitamins and there will be little or no draining off of hot water when it's time to pack your vegetables into plastic storage bags for freezing. Fresh ginger root, fresh garlic, chopped chives, and green onion stems can be stored in the freezer.

You can freeze summer melon for winter fruit salads. Cut the melon into one-inch cubes or use a melon baller. When you prepare any summer fruits or melons for freezing, add several tablespoons of fresh orange or grapefruit juice to help keep the colors bright.

Watermelon—that refreshing summer cooler—has been just as misunderstood as the much maligned potato. Far from being high-calorie, watermelon is a low-density fruit. When you consider that you can eat a whole cupful of watermelon for 175 calories and take in a good amount of fiber, iron, potassium, and three grams of protein, you are getting a bargain. All fruits contain sugar, but it's much better to get the sugar along with all the nutrients of watermelon and other fresh fruits than from refined sugar.

Dehydration is another method that enables you to prepare any fresh fruit or vegetable for storage. Like the microwave oven, the dehydrator is inexpensive to operate because it uses small amounts of electricity.

You don't have to add enhancers to dehydrated fruits and vegetables, and preparation is very easy. You needn't add preservatives or treat the food in any way. All you do is slice, dice, or chop the food. Dehydrated vegetables can be used for making soups during cold months, and when you make your own soup from scratch, you need add little salt.

Vitamins are retained in foods by dehydration. Even though the dehydration process is slow, the heat is low—only 110° to 120° F.

If you haven't had a high opinion of vegetables, fruits, and grains, change your mind. The more you explore the low-density way to eat, the easier you'll find it is to lose weight without being hungry.

Low-Density Food Enhancers

There are many easy ways to make low-density food look beautiful. Black sesame seeds (available where Oriental foods are sold) are decorative on grains and vegetables. Pieces of pimento dress up salads. A dash of red paprika or orange turmeric adds eye appeal.

Taste enhancers are vital if you are going to change your eating habits.

Fruit pulp can be used instead of sugar. You can prepare a sauce with the consistency of apple sauce from nearly any fruit by cutting the fruit into small pieces and steaming, stewing, or baking. When the fruit is tender, purée it in a blender or grinder. If you use water in cooking, use the cooking water in the blending.

You can use a little fruit pulp on bread or cereal.

Try cooking your corn or oats along with the fruit pulp. You get a mild fruit-flavored sweetness added to the grains.

Or, for a different flavor, use tea instead of water when you cook your cereal. I learned this taste trick from the Sherpas in Nepal. A favorite Sherpa dish is *tsampa*—ground wheat cooked with tea instead of water. The consistency is like mashed potatoes. Sherpas put hot chili sauce on top of their *tsampa*. You may try it with yogurt, fruit pulp, or vegetables as a topping.

Instead of a fat spread, put a little nonfat yogurt or cottage cheese on bread or toast.

Instead of salt, use soy sauce. This contains salt but only one-fifth as much as the same amount of table salt. Soy adds flavor in addition to saltiness.

Besides salt substitutes, flavor-enhancing herbs, spices, citrus juices and peels, wine, and vinegar are tasty and useful. When you cook with wine, the alcohol boils off, leaving only the flavor. Most of the calories are lost this way.

If you like hot chili, you can make your own chili sauce to enhance vegetables, grains, and cereals (see page 174).

A twist of orange or lemon peel is a flavor enhancer for tea, vegetables, or soup.

Flavor coffee New Orleans style with chicory or a tablespoonful of orange juice. To give coffee a Middle Eastern flavor, add a bit of cardamom.

If you are a tea drinker, try jasmine and other flavors of oriental tea. If you use powdered tea, to three ounces of powder add a teaspoonful of any mixture of cinnamon, powdered cloves, ginger, nutmeg, and mace. Mix very thoroughly. If you must have a tiny bit of sweetness in your tea, try this trick: use a half-teaspoon of commercial artificially sweetened tea mix and a half-teaspoon of your own spiced tea, plain powder, or lemon-flavored tea powder.

A small amount of artificial sweetener is safe. More will only feed your sweet tooth. Try to rise above this temptation.

Flavor Enhancers

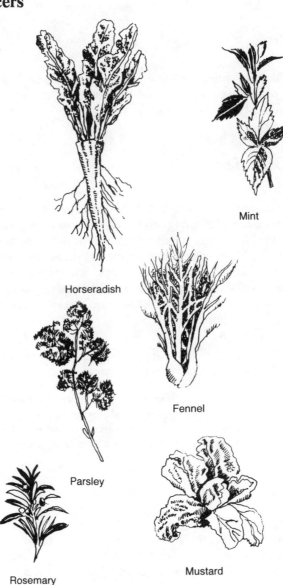

Allspice
Caraway seeds
Cardamom
Celery leaves
Chives
Cinnamon
Cloves
Coriander
Fennel
Garlic
Ginger
Horseradish
Lemon juice
Mace
Marjoram
Mint
Mustard
Nutmeg
Onion
Parsley
Pepper and chili
Poppy seeds
Rosemary
Sesame seeds
Thyme
Turmeric
Vinegar
Wine

Mint

Horseradish

Fennel

Parsley

Rosemary

Mustard

12

Meal Suggestions

Deciding what foods to eat at various times of day is often puzzling. Breakfast, especially, poses food-selection problems because of the high-sugar, high-fat customs.

Breakfast

First, don't skip breakfast. You are asking for hypoglycemia and endangering your goal of eating new foods in new ways. A good hearty breakfast with some high-protein foods will get you through the morning without longing for foods that urge you to eat more. Protein takes a long time to digest, so your pancreas need make only small and gradual amounts of insulin. If you like sweets in the morning, confine yourself to fruit or the minimum amount of sugar to sweeten your coffee or tea or a small amount of sugar substitute. Here are some possibilities:

> Fresh fruit in season or mixtures of fresh and frozen fruit (unsweetened) or stewed, dehydrated fruit.
> Hot, cooked cereal; oats, whole-wheat cereal, corn (hominy) grits, rolled barley, and wheat germ cook very fast and are very high in protein. (The more you mix grains, the more complete your protein will be.)
> Egg white cooked with vegetables or with cooked beans or bean sprouts.
> Nonfat yogurt or other nonfat milk products.

Lunch

Don't skip lunch. If you can't find a restaurant convenient to work where you can have a salad and fruit for lunch, take lunch from home. You can pack sliced raw vegetables and fruit as well as sandwiches. A slice of whole-wheat bread with yogurt may appeal to you; if you can refrigerate your lunch, take along four ounces of nonfat yogurt in a jar. This should be your basic plan:

> Salad or nonfat yogurt or other nonfat milk product
> Whole-wheat bread
> Raw vegetables cut into sticks or strips
> Fresh fruit in season

Dinner

For dinner, get into the vegetables and grains habit. Fill up to fight the night-eating syndrome.

Dinner should be your lowest density meal on ordinary days because you need less food energy in the evening when you are not working. You lose fewer calories from body-heat loss in the evening when you are home, warm and cozy, and then later tucked into your warm bed. Remember that you can eat a large, filling volume of low-density vegetables with a small calorie impact. Choose from:

> Vegetables, either cooked or raw, in salads
> Grains, either whole or ground into cereal (meaning fast-cooking) but with
>   all parts of grain left
> Fresh corn—serve with a big salad
> Fish or chicken on the weekend

You may know by now that there is no vegetable on earth that cannot be put in a salad. Remember when buying grains that most commercial corn grits are degerminated. Get ground, whole corn if you can; it's very nutritious. Keep it in the refrigerator or freezer.

Corn is a high-protein grain. And if you add cooked beans or fresh, raw bean sprouts to your salad, you will have completed the protein of your meal (bean sprouts add amino acids).

Vary the seasonings and herbs on your fish and chicken and the types of vegetables you serve with them. Make your dinner a beautiful event by adding colorful herbs, spices, and garnishes.

Dessert

Eat fruit for dessert, if you must have dessert. Be sure to fill up on low-density cooked and raw vegetables at dinnertime to help you forget food until morning.

LOW-DENSITY RECIPES

It is important to remember that you are embarking on a new way of eating; it may take some time for you to stop wanting old favorites and to acquire new eating habits and pleasures. To start you on your way to eating for better health, here are a few sample menu suggestions and recipes. They should stir your imagination in the right direction. Don't be afraid to improvise on them to suit your needs, based on your own food tastes. Directions given here are for conventional range cookery, but most of the recipes can be adapted to a microwave oven, pressure cooker, or a slow cooker by following the manufacturer's directions. The recipes can easily be doubled and even tripled in most cases to feed family and friends.

You can get inspiration and ideas as well as specific recipes from the many specialty cookbooks on the market today. "Organic," "natural foods," "health foods," "vegetarian," and "whole-grain" are some of the clue words in your treasure hunt. Books specializing in the cuisine of the Orient, the Middle East, India, Latin America, and other faraway places can be excellent sources for new dishes. Just keep in mind the principles of low-density cookery, and when you use other cookbooks, remember to make the following modifications: Cut back the amount of or eliminate oils and animal fats, dried fruits and nuts, honey, sugar, and molasses. Think "low density," think "vegetables," and think "grains." Turn away from meats and sweets and all such high-density problem foods.

Breakfast: Suggested Menus

Orange slices with cinnamon   Broiled pear slices*
Rice-millet cereal*   Ricotta or pot cheese
Beverage   Beverage

*Recipe follows.

Fresh grapefruit   Fresh strawberries
Egg scramble*   Baked farmer cheese*
Beverage   Beverage

                                     Vegetable cocktail*
                                     Three-grain cereal*
                                     Beverage

Rice-Millet Cereal

2½ cups water or skim milk   ½ cup rice
⅛ teaspoon salt substitute†   ½ cup millet

In a medium saucepan, bring water or skim milk and salt substitute to a
boil. Stir in rice and millet. Cover; simmer until liquid is absorbed, about 35
to 40 minutes. Makes 2 servings.

Egg Scramble

2 egg whites   1 scallion stem, chopped
⅓–½ cup bean sprouts   Dash of soy sauce

In a small bowl, beat all ingredients well with a fork. Pour mixture into
a small skillet (either Teflon-type, or lightly coated with non-stick vegetable spray). Over low heat, scramble mixture lightly with fork until cooked,
about 3 minutes. Serve with another dash of soy sauce, if desired. Makes 1
serving.

Broiled Pear Slices

1 fresh pear   Freshly grated nutmeg or cinnamon

Wash and core pear, but do not pare; cut in eighths. Place pear slices in
a single layer in a ramekin or small baking dish (a small foil pan works very
well). Sprinkle generously with nutmeg. Cook under preheated broiler until
heated through and juices appear, about 7 to 10 minutes. Makes 1 serving.

Baked Farmer Cheese

4 ounces skim-milk farmer cheese   Freshly grated nutmeg or cinnamon
¼ teaspoon grated orange rind

Lightly flatten and shape farmer cheese into a patty; place in a small
ramekin or baking dish; sprinkle with orange rind. Cook under preheated
broiler until lightly golden or puffed, about 5 to 7 minutes. Sprinkle generously with nutmeg. Makes 1 serving.

---

†Use Lite-salt, or one of the many salt substitutes on the market.

Vegetable Cocktail

1 cup vegetable broth††
1 tomato, peeled
½ carrot, chopped

½ bell pepper, seeded and chopped
Dash of tabasco sauce

In blender container, whirl all ingredients until liquid is as smooth as possible, about 1½ to 2 minutes. Chill before serving. Makes 1 serving. (This is an excellent between-meals' pick-me-up. On a hot summer day, blend with three ice cubes; or heat cocktail for a cold-weather warmer.)

Three-Grain Cereal

1¼ cups water
2 ounces old-fashioned oats

2 ounces corn grits (hominy)
2 ounces wheat germ

In a small saucepan, bring water to a boil. Stir in grains in order given; lower heat and continue cooking, stirring constantly, until water is absorbed, about 5 minutes. Take off heat; cover; let stand five minutes before serving.

Lunch: Suggested Menus

Spinach salad*
Orange
Beverage

Minestrone soup*
Plum
Beverage

Slaw salad*
Slice of whole wheat bread
Beverage

Eggplant salad*
Cherry tomatoes, carrot slices
Beverage

Three-bean salad*
Strawberries
Beverage

Chicken-stuffed zucchini*
Banana
Beverage

Creamy bean spread*
Tomato, carrot, and zucchini slices
Beverage
Green pepper and carrot sticks

Sweet and spicy bean spread*
Apple and pear slices
Beverage

Cottage cheese and yogurt
Green beans with cumin*
Nectarine
Beverage

Mixed vegetable salad*
Slice of whole wheat bread
Pear
Beverage

††Save and refrigerate or freeze the liquid that remains after steaming vegetables; use the liquid as cooking broth.
*Recipe follows.

Spinach Salad

4 cups fresh spinach leaves
¼ pound mushrooms, sliced
1 cup nonfat or low-fat yogurt
1 teaspoon lemon juice
1 clove garlic, minced

1 teaspoon fresh dill (or ½ teaspoon
  dried dillweed)
1 cup cooked white beans
Freshly ground pepper

Wash and dry spinach. Place spinach and mushrooms in serving dish; toss. In a small bowl, combine yogurt, lemon juice, garlic and dill; stir in white beans. Spoon mixture into center of spinach; chill. Just before serving, add pepper to taste and toss salad. Makes 2 servings.

Slaw Salad

2 cups shredded cabbage
½ cup diced celery
½ cup grated carrot
1 medium apple, chopped

1 tablespoon raisins
¾ cup yogurt
2 tablespoons orange juice
Chicory

In a medium bowl, combine all ingredients except chicory; stir well; chill. At serving time, spoon onto chicory. Makes 2 servings.

Three-Bean Salad

½ cup cooked kidney beans
½ cup cooked chick peas
½ cup cooked green beans
½ cup cooked corn
¼ cup chopped green pepper
½ Bermuda onion, thinly sliced

1 tablespoon minced radish
¼ cup wine vinegar
¼ teaspoon paprika
⅛ teaspoon salt substitute†
Romaine

In a medium bowl, combine all ingredients except romaine; stir well. Let stand at room temperature, stirring several times, for 30 minutes; chill. At serving time, spoon bean salad onto romaine. Sprinkle with additional paprika, if desired. Makes 2 servings.

Creamy Bean Spread

1 cup cooked chick peas
½ cup cooked kidney beans
½ cup cooked lentils

1 clove garlic, minced
½–1 teaspoon lemon juice
¼ teaspoon turmeric

Run legumes through food mill or whirl in a blender; spoon into a medium bowl. Stir in remaining ingredients; chill. Spread on thin slices of raw vegetable such as turnip, carrot, rutabaga, cucumber, cauliflower, or tomato. Makes 4 servings.

†Use Lite-salt, or one of the many salt substitutes on the market.

Green Beans with Cumin

½ pound green beans, washed and tipped
⅛ teaspoon salt substitute†
¼ teaspoon dry mustard
1 teaspoon ground cumin

1 tablespoon minced shallots or onion
2 tablespoons wine vinegar
Freshly ground pepper to taste

Steam beans until just tender, about 10 minutes. Drain; place in serving dish. In a small bowl, mix together all remaining ingredients with a wire whisk. Pour the vinegar mixture over the warm beans and toss well. Serve at once. Makes 2 servings.

Minestrone Soup

½ cup mixed dried legumes (chick peas, pinto, lima, white beans, etc.)
4 tomatoes, fresh or canned
1 leek or onion, chopped
1 cup celery tops, chopped
2 cloves garlic, minced
¼ cup chopped parsley

½ teaspoon oregano, crushed
1 teaspoon lemon juice
3 quarts vegetable broth†† or water
Freshly ground pepper to taste
4 cups mixed vegetables (corn, zucchini, green beans, mushrooms, escarole, etc.)

In a large kettle, place all ingredients except for the 4 cups of mixed vegetables. Bring to a boil; cover; simmer for 1 hour. Stir in the mixed vegetables; cover; simmer for another hour. Ladle into soup bowls and top with additional chopped parsley, if desired. Makes 4 to 6 servings.

Eggplant Salad

1 small eggplant (about 1 pound)
1 clove garlic, minced
⅛ teaspoon salt substitute†

1 small onion, finely chopped
1–2 tablespoons lemon juice to taste

Wash and wipe eggplant; prick all over with fork. Place eggplant on a baking sheet in cold oven. Turn oven to 500 degrees and bake eggplant 30 minutes; turn eggplant over and bake 20 minutes longer. Remove from oven and let it cool just enough to handle. In a medium bowl, mash garlic and salt substitute with a wooden spoon. Hold eggplant over the bowl; slit skin and scrape pulp into the bowl. Discard skin. Stir in remaining ingredients. Chill several hours before serving. Makes 2 servings.

†Use Lite-salt, or one of the many salt substitutes on the market.
††Save and refrigerate or freeze the liquid that remains after steaming vegetables; use the liquid as cooking broth.

Chicken-Stuffed Zucchini

2 medium zucchini, cooked and sliced
   lengthwise
1 cup shredded cooked chicken
½ cup chopped cooked carrot
½ cup sliced raw mushrooms

1 small tomato, chopped
1 tablespoon chopped scallion stem
2 tablespoons white wine
2 tablespoons tarragon vinegar

Scoop out zucchini pulp and place in a medium bowl, setting shells aside. Stir in remaining ingredients, mixing well. With a spoon, mound mixture into zucchini shells. Chill well before serving. Makes 2 servings.

Sweet and Spicy Bean Spread

1 cup cooked white beans
½ cup cooked kidney beans
½ cup cooked chick peas
1 tablespoon orange juice

1 teaspoon grated orange rind
¼ teaspoon each of ground clove, nutmeg, and cinnamon

Run legumes through food mill or whirl in blender until smooth; spoon into a medium bowl. Stir in remaining ingredients; chill. To serve, spread on thin slices of raw fruit such as melon, apple, pear, or orange. Makes 4 servings.

Mixed Vegetable Salad

2 cooked carrots
3 cooked new (red) potatoes
3 cooked beets
1 Bermuda onion

½ cup nonfat or low-fat cottage cheese
1 tablespoon minced radish
¼ teaspoon dill seed
Watercress

Dice carrots and potatoes; slice beets and onion. Stir lightly in a medium bowl to combine vegetables. In a small bowl, stir together cottage cheese, radish, and dill seed. To serve, spoon vegetables onto watercress; top with cottage cheese mixture. Makes 2 servings.

Dinner: Suggested Menus

Salad greens tossed with yogurt and
   dill
Sherpa stew*
Beverage

Company fish stew*
Salad bowl
Crusty rolls
Beverage

Soy Chicken*
Rice cooked with bean sprouts and
   water chestnuts
Spinach with sesame seeds
Beverage

Grated carrot and pineapple salad
Vegetable goulash*
Kasha
Beverage

*Recipes follow.

Tomato, carrot, and green pepper slices
Yam and peas*
Beverage

Cucumber with yogurt and chopped mint
Spinach and bulgar*
Beverage

Ceviche*
Artichoke hearts cooked with sliced carrots
Beverage

Tomato aspic
Kale and rice*
Beverage

Vegetable kebabs*
Rice
Corn-on-the-cob
Beverage

Potato cress supper soup*
Baked acorn squash
Fruit crush*
Beverage

Sherpa Stew

1 large potato, scrubbed but not pared

1 bunch mustard greens
Chili Sauce

Dice potato in ½-inch cubes; place in steamer and cook until barely soft, about 10 minutes. Cut mustard greens into 1-inch pieces; add to potato; continue cooking until vegetables are tender, about 5 minutes. Serve with Chili Sauce. Makes 1 serving.

Chili Sauce

Cut up two fresh or canned tomatoes and Jalapeno pepper to taste; add ¼ cup water. Whirl in a blender just long enough to blend ingredients into a sauce. Or: Whirl tomato and water with a little chopped onion, sweet bell pepper, and a dash of tabasco sauce. Makes ½ cup.

Soy Chicken

2 pounds chicken parts
4 teaspoons soy sauce

½ teaspoon ground ginger
1 clove garlic, minced

Rinse chicken and pat dry. Cut away and discard all visible fat. In a small bowl, stir together remaining ingredients; rub mixture into chicken. Place chicken in a casserole; cover; cook in preheated 350-degree oven until tender, about 1¼ hours. Remove casserole from oven; drain chicken on paper towel; set aside, but keep warm. (You may remove skin at this point to further reduce fat content and still have moist, succulent meat.) Pour juices from casserole into freezer container; chill in freezer until fat rises to top, about 15 minutes; skim off fat and discard. Reheat remaining juices and serve over chicken. Makes 6 servings.

Yam and Peas

1 large yam or sweet potato, scrubbed but not pared	*⅓ cup green peas* *Fresh mint (optional)*

Steam or bake potato until barely soft, about 30 to 40 minutes. Lightly steam peas until just barely cooked, about 5 minutes; drain well, reserving juices in steamer. Dice potato into a small bowl; mash with fork until as smooth as possible; place in steamer. Spoon peas on top of potato; cover; steam until peas are tender and potato is heated through, about 5 minutes. Serve with fresh mint to taste. Makes 1 serving.

Ceviche

1 pound lean white fish fillets (turbot, sole, haddock, etc.)
2 ounces fresh lime juice (from about 4 limes)
2 medium tomatoes, peeled and chopped
½ Jalapeno pepper, chopped, or
tabasco sauce to taste
1 small onion, finely chopped
1 tablespoon chopped cilantro (coriander) or parsley
½ teaspoon oregano, crushed
1 tablespoon white wine
2 tablespoons vinegar

Cut fish into bite-size pieces. Place in a small glass dish (do not use metal). Pour lime juice over fish; marinate for 1½ hours, turning fish several times. In medium skillet, over low heat, poach fish in the lime juice, just until bubbles begin to form at edge of skillet (add about ¼ cup water if necessary). Remove from heat; cover and let stand to cool slightly, about 10 minutes. Drain fish well; place in serving dish. Add remaining ingredients; stir lightly, just to combine with fish. Chill before serving. Makes 2 servings.

NOTE: Stuffed into mushroom buttons, Ceviche makes an elegant party hors d'ouevre.

Vegetable Kebabs

¼ cup soy sauce
¼ cup sake (white wine)
1 teaspoon ginger
1 clove garlic, minced
2 tomatoes, quartered
1 green pepper, cubed
4 small white onions
1 zucchini, sliced in 1-inch pieces
8 mushroom caps

In medium bowl, stir together the first four ingredients. Add the vegetables to soy mixture; marinate, stirring several times, for 2 to 3 hours at room temperature. Remove vegetables from marinade and thread on two skewers. Broil in the oven or barbecue, basting often with the marinade, until the kebabs are tender and well-browned, about 15 to 20 minutes. Remove from skewers and serve on top of hot rice. Makes 2 servings.

Company Fish Stew

6 medium tomatoes, chopped
2 medium potatoes, chopped
1 large onion, chopped
2 cloves garlic, minced
2 tablespoons chopped parsley
¼ teaspoon thyme, crushed
¼ teaspoon marjoram, crushed
½ teaspoon saffron, crushed
1 bay leaf
1 cup tomato juice

1 cup clam broth
2 cups white wine
2 cups vegetable broth†† or water
1 pound lean white fish fillets (turbot,
   haddock, etc.)
1 dozen clams, scrubbed
½ pound medium-size shrimp, peeled
   and deveined
½ pound scallops

In a kettle, stir together all ingredients except the fish and shellfish. Cover; simmer 30 minutes. Remove bay leaf; add remaining ingredients. Cover; simmer another 20 to 30 minutes. Serve in soup bowls. Makes 6 to 8 servings.

Vegetable Goulash

1 quart vegetable broth†† or water
2 tablespoons red or white wine
1 clove garlic, minced
1 tablespoon chopped parsley (or 1
   teaspoon dried flakes)
1 teaspoon chopped basil (or ½ teaspoon dried basil, crushed)
⅛ teaspoon salt substitute†
¼ teaspoon freshly ground pepper
2 cups shredded cabbage

2 cups shredded romaine
2 kohlrabi bulbs
1 large rutabaga
1 medium onion
½ green pepper, seeded
¼ pound peas, including tipped
   pods
6 mushrooms
2 large tomatoes

In a kettle, mix the vegetable broth or water, wine, garlic, parsley, basil, salt substitute, and pepper. Add cabbage and lettuce. Cover; simmer until vegetables have wilted and cooked down, about 15 minutes. Dice remaining ingredients into the kettle; stir well. Cover; simmer until vegetables are tender and most of the liquid is absorbed, about 2½ to 3 hours. Serve in soup plates. Makes 4 servings.

Spinach and Bulgar

½ cup fine bulgar
Water
1 medium onion, chopped
1 pound spinach, finely chopped,

washed, and lightly drained
⅛ teaspoon salt substitute†
Juice of 1 lemon

Soak bulgar in one cup of cold water for 15 minutes; drain. In a medium skillet (Teflon or lightly coated with non-stick vegetable spray), over low heat,

†Use Lite-salt, or one of the many salt substitutes on the market.
††Save and refrigerate or freeze the liquid that remains after steaming vegetables; use the liquid as cooking broth.

cook onion until soft, adding a teaspoon or two of water if necessary. Add spinach with whatever water is still clinging to it; stir until tender and most of moisture is absorbed, about 5 minutes. Add bulgar and salt substitute; stir until well mixed with spinach mixture and heated through, about 5 minutes. Add lemon juice just before serving. Makes 2 servings.

Kale and Rice

1 cup finely chopped kale, washed,   ⅓ cup white rice
   and lightly drained   ⅓ cup brown rice
2 scallions, chopped   2 cups fat-free chicken broth
1 carrot, grated   Mace

In a medium saucepan, combine all ingredients except mace. Bring to a boil; lower heat, cover and simmer until liquid is absorbed, about 25 to 35 minutes. Just before serving, dust with mace. Makes 2 servings.

Potato Cress Supper Soup

2 medium potatoes, scrubbed but not   ½ cup skim milk
   pared   ½ cup nonfat or low-fat yogurt
Potato water   Salt substitute†
1 onion, chopped   Freshly ground pepper
1 bunch watercress, chopped

In a medium saucepan, boil potatoes until soft, about 20 minutes. Measure and set aside 1 cup of the cooking water; dice potatoes. In a large saucepan, over low heat, cook the onion in its own juices until soft, about 3 minutes. (Add a tablespoon of water, if necessary, to keep from sticking.) Stir in potato, potato water, and watercress; cover; simmer 5 minutes. Add milk, yogurt, salt substitute, and ground pepper to taste. Heat soup, but do not boil. Ladle into soup bowls. Makes 2 servings.

Fruit Crush

3 or 4 ice cubes   1 banana, sliced
1 grapefruit, sectioned and chilled   Fresh chopped mint (optional)

Place ice cubes in blender; cover; whirl long enough to crush ice, about 30 seconds. Flicking blender on and off, add grapefruit a few sections at a time; whirl just until mixture turns to an icy consistency, about 15 seconds. Add banana a few slices at a time; whirl just until mixture is a thick snowy consistency, about ½ to 1 minute. Serve in a tall glass with a bit of mint, if desired. Makes 1 serving. (This makes an excellent between-meal appetite appeaser and can help fight off a demoralizing eating binge.)

†Use Lite-salt, or one of the many salt substitutes on the market.

SUGGESTIONS FOR SINGLES

Many singles are in the habit of grabbing something to eat when they're hungry. The worst part of this bad habit is that the food is often junk food.

You owe it to yourself and to your self-esteem to make your encounters with food as healthy and weight-conscious as possible. Your weight and your health are just as important as your career, your job, and your personal goals. Make eating an important part of your life and you.

All you need to do is to set some standards for yourself about eating and food habits and stick to them. It's as easy as brushing your teeth.

Make a contract with yourself to plan all your food for each day. During periods when you're very busy and don't want to be bothered, eat the same thing every day and save up to have fancier foods on the weekend.

Plan all your food and eating for the week. Shop with a list and stick to it. Buy your week's supply of food on one shopping trip. Vow not to let anything lower your sales resistance to high-calorie high-density food.

If you hate to cook or don't have time, that's fine. You can have excellent, nourishing, low-calorie, filling meals with simple grains, fresh fruits and vegetables, dried beans and legumes, and nonfat milk products.

Many singles skip breakfast. It's a bad habit whatever your reasons may be. Oatmeal, corn grits, and whole-wheat cereal are fast and easy to prepare. The smartest kind of instant breakfast is a bowl of hot cereal, cooked for two minutes in a microwave oven. You cook and eat the cereal in the same dish. If this method is not for you, whole-grain cereal cooked in the usual way is sensational for providing natural flavor, hunger satisfaction, and nutritional benefits. Because it's hot, you have to eat it more slowly than cold cereal, even if you cool it a bit with fruit or yogurt. When you eat slowly, your fullness feelings come on better than when you eat fast. When you have to cook your food, even if the cooking method is fast, you're less likely to fill up your bowl again. Fresh fruit cut up in the cereal adds a little sweetness and adds fiber to your diet. An orange can be peeled and cut up in less than two minutes.

Take your lunch to work, and on days when you go out for lunch, order a big salad.

If you find you feel better when you nibble, take raw-vegetable snacks to work. Eat two or three carrots and a turnip or two at your morning and afternoon breaks. Cut them into thin sticks. They're clean, they won't mess your hands, they taste good, and they're very satisfying. They also have anticonstipating fiber.

When you come home exhausted after a hard day's work, a dinner of oatmeal and corn or wheat cereal is faster to prepare than a TV dinner. Eat it with raw vegetables. You can't eat raw vegetables fast; they take too long to chew. Drink water or nonfat milk and sip and munch slowly. Read a book with your evening meal. Even if the meal takes an hour, you will be relaxed and full. Have a piece of fresh fruit for dessert. After a meal like this, you'll be ready to forget about eating till the next day.

On the weekend, you can try your hand at more involved foods made from scratch. (See the chicken recipe on page 174, for example.) You can prepare and freeze individual portions of chicken or other foods in plastic bags. Take out a portion during the week when you want a change of menu.

On the weekend, invite a guest or two to a dinner party. If you like to cook, make a hobby out of cooking the low-density way.

SNACKS AND EATING OUT

A banana is a good snack. It's the highest-protein fruit, and bananas are filling and nutritious.

In summer, try snacks of melon. Cut off the rind and slice the fruit into finger-length pieces. Cantaloupe, watermelon, honeydew, and casaba are among the best low-density fruits; you get a large volume and few calories.

Pears and apples are good snack foods. Pears are lower in density than apples but the extra thirty or so calories are insignificant unless you binge. Grapefruit sections are another fine snack food. If you need a taste enhancer, sprinkle the sections with cinnamon, ginger, mace, or nutmeg. You can also broil the sections for five minutes or heat them in a microwave oven for two minutes.

Raw-vegetable snacks are the lowest-calorie, most colorful and crunchiest nibbling foods of all. For parties, try cutting shapes out of turnip slices with cooky cutters. Beets scrubbed and sliced make colorful party snacks. Cucumber and zucchini add variety. Shaped vegetable slices stuck on toothpicks and set into a whole grapefruit or a bowl made of half a watermelon are tempting. You can fill the rest of the "bowl" with cauliflowerets, broccoli buds, carrot sticks, radishes, small celery sticks, and sprigs of parsley. You'll never miss crackers and pretzels once you become acquainted with vegetable hors d'oeuvres.

Mushroom buttons, stuffed with grated carrot or radish marinated in wine vinegar or with equal amounts of nonfat cottage cheese and canned minced clams, are delicious. The same mix, made thinner, can be used as a dip. Freshly chopped chives, oregano, parsley, onion, or chili sauce can be used to add flavor.

Plain puffed wheat and puffed rice are good snack foods. Other plain, puffed grains that have recently become available in the food markets are corn and millet.

A study showed that overweight children accept raw vegetables and fresh fruit as substitutes for junk food. The important thing was that the snack, to be identified as such, had to be small enough to be picked up with the fingers. If overweight children will accept healthy low-calorie snacks, overweight adults should be able to do so.

Afternoon hours, especially around four o'clock, are a time of jitters and hypoglycemia. Tea and vegetable snacks or fresh fruit solve this problem.

Evenings with friends in a restaurant are a challenge to many people. Drink tea, grapefruit juice, or tomato juice if you do not want to feel left out. If you are really hungry late at night, order a small dinner salad along with your tea or juice.

Beverages often pose a problem for weight-conscious people. Do not turn to bouillon. It is high in salt. Instead, try any of numerous teas—herb teas and tea blends—to help fill that empty feeling without the impact of salt or calories. Above all, develop an appreciation for water.

Restaurant eating as a whole is a problem. When you order salad in a restaurant, always ask to have your dressing on the side so you can use small, restrained amounts of these high-calorie, high-salt preparations. When you order a baked potato in a restaurant, always ask for it to be dry, without butter or sour cream. Teach yourself to prefer the natural goodness of baked potato without greasy, high-density enhancers. Some restaurants will be happy to serve you plain chopped chives on the side for your baked potato.

When you are faced with high-density food in a restaurant where you have no choice, leave food over. Trim meats well, chew each bite at least twenty times, and never eat the gravy. If you can stop after eating one French fry, eat one, but only one. If fish or seafood are breaded, cut the greasy breading away.

Large-appetite, low-density eaters usually can be satisfied with soup and salad. If the menu doesn't have these choices, relax, be sociable, choose the lowest-calorie alternative, and vow to cut down the next day. Being as prudent as you can in a social situation will help you learn to make choices —realize that your friends will feel uncomfortable if you eat nothing; so face reality and do the best you can.

Traveling is relatively easy on an airplane where food portions are small, but cruises, train trips and traveling long distances by car can make eating complex.

Look for restaurants with salad bars or with buffets that offer many vegetable and salad selections. These are springing up throughout the country. Buy fresh fruit at a grocery store and prepare your own breakfast at a hotel or motel. Opt for restaurants where you can choose not to have foods covered with fat, sauces, and sugar. Order a la carte to avoid any confrontations with rich desserts. Drink water while waiting for your food to be served instead of being tempted by crackers or rolls. When you can limit yourself to one plain roll without butter, eat it very slowly, a tiny bite at a time. In other countries, stick to fish and cooked vegetables and fruits. I have been successful at buying fresh fruit in market stalls as far away as in Nepal and India. My secret is to take the fruits back to the hotel and wash them thoroughly with hot water and hand soap before eating them. Try the native cooking, but avoid all added fats. Remember what you learn from the Break the Rules Calorie Counter: mixtures of meat, fat, and grains or flour are very high-density foods. They average 200 calories in 6 tablespoons. Above all, when traveling, exercise as much as you can.

People who have developed a long-term commitment, about a year or longer, to low-density, high-volume eating have a hard time at a fast-food chain. Their tastes have changed. Hamburgers, ribs, and fried chicken taste greasy to them. Milk-shakes, ice cream, malts, and desserts become unbearably sweet.

Your ultimate goal is to learn to eat to live. Wherever you are, whatever you are doing, work at making the event of the meal, the company, and the surroundings at least as important as the food.

SUGGESTIONS FOR BREAKING THE RULES

If you learn how to follow the rules of low-density eating, you will be so pleased with your weight loss that you may not want to break the rules.

There are all sorts of little things you can do to enhance lean, simple low-density food. One recipe that breaks the rules starts with a dry powdered commercial packaged salad dressing that is high in salt, called low-calorie salad dressing. It has the advantage of being prepared with acacia. Acacia is a harmless plant product that helps thicken the sauce without using fat. Adding a large amount of tomato juice dilutes the salt. The final salad dressing has an insignificant amount of salt in each portion.

Another rule breaker is pouring any leftover wine into your vinegar to enhance the flavor. The calories you add will not be significant, and the wine will soon turn to vinegar.

All meats contain marbled fat. It's impossible to get rid of all the fat. When you want to break the rules and eat high-density protein, there are three things that will decrease the amount of fat you get. Buy the cheapest cuts of meat; these have the least marbling, but the meat may be tough and stringy. To get around the toughness, the meat may be sliced or ground. Slice the cheap cuts into very thin pieces so they can be chewed, or grind cheap cuts that have been carefully trimmed of all visible fat.

With the ground meat, you can prepare meat sauces, meat patties, or meatballs, although the density will still be much higher than fish or chicken or vegetable protein. With the slices you can prepare teriyaki or meat and vegetable mixtures.

To break the rules, see the Break the Rules Calorie Counter on page 222. All the typical high-density foods are listed: pizza, desserts, and so on. Each food is given in the portion size that contains 200 calories. When you get ready to break the rules, this special-occasion calorie-counter list will come in handy.

Set some standards for yourself for when and how to break the rules. Here are some tips:

A Lifetime Weight Expert's Guide to Breaking the Rules

Ice cream: 1 scoop on your birthday (if chocolate or a nut flavor, only ½ scoop).

Chocolate: 2 pieces of chocolate a year, on Christmas or on your most important holiday.

Cake: 1 piece, once a year, at a very special person's wedding.

Hard candy: Never.

Soda pop: 2 sips on the hottest day of the year, if there is no pure water within five blocks.

Olives: 2, once a year (green or black, the density and calorie impact are the same)

Bacon: Never.

Pizza: 1 medium-sized slice twice a year.

Barbecued ribs: One rib a year after you have been at your ideal weight for five years and if you vow to walk five miles after licking the grease off your fingers.

Hot cakes and syrup: 2 small cakes once a year on your vacation; no butter or margarine is allowed, but you can have 1 tablespoon of syrup or 1 teaspoon of jam or jelly.

Danish, Viennese, or French pastry: ½ portion once a year on a special occasion.

Steak: 1 small one, well done, once a month, followed by a five-mile walk.

French fries and potato chips: Never, unless you can stop after eating just one.

Sausage: Never, unless you can stop after one bite.

Do you want to be at your ideal weight for your lifetime? The road to success is hard at first, but I assure you it gets easier after a while. You have to assert yourself. There is no magic to it, and no one else can do it for you.

You have to make your own decision to have complete, conscious control every time you are confronted with food.

When you have that control, you will find that you will like yourself.

GLOSSARY

ANOREXIA NERVOSA   A serious appetite disturbance found in teenagers; although more common in girls, anorexia nervosa occurs in boys also. These young people *will* not to eat; the condition is very difficult to treat.

ARTERIOSCLEROSIS   Hardening of small arteries caused by gradual building up of cholesterol deposits over the years.

ATHEROSCLEROSIS   The same condition as arteriosclerosis, occurring in larger arteries.

ATHEROSCLEROTIC HEART DISEASE   Weakness and decreased function of the beating action of the heart caused by poor blood supply because of atherosclerosis of the coronary arteries.

ATROPHY   Decrease in size of a part of the body due to lack of use of the part.

BOMB CALORIMETRY   The scientific method for finding out the number of calories in a food. The method is very expensive; therefore, many prepared and processed foods have their calories estimated from the calories of their components.

CELLULITE   The lumpy, flabby skin of many overweight people. This is not a medical term, but it is very appropriate to use instead of the word "flab."

CHOLESTEROL   One of the products of fat metabolism in all animals and humans. It is made in the human liver in sufficient amounts to supply all the needs for bile and hormones. It has a great tendency to form plaques on the walls of arteries, which gradually become dense and hard.

DENTAL CARIES   Decay and disintegration of teeth. Sugar has now been proven to be a leading cause.

ENDOGENOUS   Produced from within. The use in this book refers to cholesterol that is produced in the human body.

EXOGENOUS   Produced from without. The use in this book refers to cholesterol produced in the bodies of animals that are then eaten by humans. This intake adds to the total cholesterol in the human body.

GASTRITIS   Inflammation of the stomach.

GI	Stands for gastrointestinal and means the human digestive system.
GLUCOSE	A simple sugar consisting of one molecule and very important in human metabolism. The sugar in the human body is glucose.
HIGH-VOLUME FOODS	Foods that are high in bulk and low in calories.
HYPERTROPHY	Enlargement of part of the body due to use and activity of the part.
HYPERLIPIDEMIA	A condition of the human body consisting of persistently high blood cholesterol (220 milligrams* or more) and blood fat (140 milligrams or more).
HYPOGLYCEMIA	A low level of glucose in the blood. The level at which adrenalin is produced and symptoms are felt varies from person to person. The level at which adrenalin is produced and symptoms are felt in any individual is changeable and varies with weight gain and loss, and the condition of the person's metabolism.
IRON-DEFICIENCY ANEMIA	A deficiency in the red blood cells caused by a lack of sufficient iron in the body.
ISOMETRIC EXERCISE	Exercise done by contracting muscles while the body is not moving. This exercise increases the flow of blood to the heart, but the heart does not increase the number of times it beats each minute, thereby elevating the blood pressure in the body.
KETOSIS	An excess of acid in the body that may be caused by starvation, fasting, diabetes, or eating excessive quantities of foods that leave acid in the body when they are metabolized.
LIPOPROTEIN	A special type of fat in the blood that transports cholesterol and blood fat from one part of the body to another via the bloodstream. When cholesterol or blood fat is elevated, lipoprotein also becomes elevated.
LOW-DENSITY FOODS	Foods with the least calories in the largest portions.
METABOLISM	The chemistry by which living cells take food energy and make their own energy to sustain life, promote growth, and carry on repair of the body cells.
MYOCARDIAL INFARCTION	Destruction and death of heart-muscle cells caused by obstruction of the coronary blood supply to a portion of heart muscle.
OSTEOPOROSIS	A painful bone condition occurring in middle life and later due to decalcification of bone. Once it occurs, there is no cure; prevention consists of exercise and

*The safeness of the cholesterol level of 220 is being seriously questioned, and the maximum is being set at under 200 by many cardiologists.

sound calcium and phosphorus nutrition in the growing and adult years of life.

PELLAGRA   A disease caused by a dietary deficiency of the vitamin B complex. It is practically unheard of in North America at this time except in chronic alcoholics.

PEPTIC ULCER   A painful erosion of the lining of the stomach or first part of the small intestine, caused in part by the corrosive action of stomach juice.

PICA   A craving for unnatural food such as chalk, dirt, or newspaper.

PHYTIC ACID   A compound present in large quantities in wheat and rice bran. Phytic acid prevents the absorption of iron by the GI tract.

SUBCUTANEOUS FAT   Fat that is deposited beneath the skin of the body and that forms part of a person's outward appearance.

TRIGLYCERIDE   The major portion of storage fat and blood fat in humans. It consists of three molecules of fatty acid attached to one molecule of glycerin.

APPENDIX

Calorie and food-composition charts are not mathematically exact. Foods differ in their composition in different parts of the world and at different times during their seasons. Absorption of nutrients varies when foods are raw or cooked. Exact calorie determinations are not done on many processed foods; they are often estimated.

1. STANDARD AMERICAN HEIGHTS AND WEIGHTS

HEIGHT	WEIGHT				
	Women			Men	
	Average	Range		Average	Range
4'10"	102	92–119			
4'11"	104	94–122			
5'0"	107	96–125			
5'1"	110	99–128			
5'2"	113	102–131		123	112–141
5'3"	116	105–134		127	115–144
5'4"	120	108–138		130	118–148
5'5"	123	111–142		133	121–152
5'6"	128	114–146		136	124–156
5'7"	132	118–150		140	128–161
5'8"	136	122–154		145	132–166
5'9"	140	126–158		149	136–170
5'10"	144	130–163		153	140–174
5'11"	148	134–168		158	144–179
6'0"	152	138–173		162	148–184
6'1"				166	152–189
6'2"				171	156–194
6'3"				176	160–199
6'4"				181	164–204

2. STANDARD AMERICAN TRICEPS SKIN FOLD MEASUREMENTS

Age (Years)	Women	Men
5	0.55118 (1.4)*	0.4724 (1.2)
6	0.59055 (1.5)	0.4724 (1.2)
7	0.62992 (1.6)	0.5118 (1.3)
8	0.66929 (1.7)	0.55118 (1.4)
9	0.70866 (1.8)	0.59055 (1.5)
10	0.78740 (2.0)	0.62992 (1.6)
11	0.82677 (2.1)	0.66929 (1.7)
12	0.86614 (2.2)	0.70866 (1.8)
13	0.90551 (2.3)	0.70866 (1.8)
14	0.90551 (2.3)	0.66929 (1.7)
15	0.94488 (2.4)	0.62992 (1.6)
16	0.98425 (2.5)	0.59055 (1.5)
17	1.02362 (2.6)	0.55118 (1.4)
18	1.06299 (2.7)	0.59055 (1.5)
19	1.06299 (2.7)	0.59055 (1.5)
20	1.10236 (2.8)	0.62992 (1.5)
21	1.10236 (2.8)	0.66929 (1.6)
22	1.10236 (2.8)	0.70866 (1.8)
23	1.10236 (2.8)	0.70866 (1.9)
24	1.10236 (2.8)	0.74803 (2.0)
25	1.14173 (2.9)	0.7874 (2.0)
26	1.14173 (2.9)	0.7874 (2.0)
27	1.14173 (2.9)	0.82677 (2.1)
28	1.14173 (2.9)	0.86614 (2.2)
29	1.14173 (2.9)	0.86614 (2.2)
30–50	1.1811 (3.0)	0.90551 (2.3)

*The decimal figure is given in inches. The figure in parentheses is given in centimeters.

3. HOW TO CALCULATE YOUR PHYSICAL FITNESS*

I. Men

START WITH TABLE I:

1. Find your body weight.
2. Locate your pulse rate in After-Exercise Pulse Rate column.
3. Opposite your pulse rate and above your age, find your fitness-index number.
4. Now go to Table II.

Table I
YOUR FITNESS-INDEX NUMBER

After-Exercise Pulse Rate										
180	5	5	5	5	5	5	5	5	5	5
170	5	5	5	5	5	5	5	5	5	5
160	5	5	5	5	5	5	5	5	5	5
150	5	5	5	4	4	4	4	4	4	4
140	4	4	4	4	4	4	4	4	4	4
130	4	4	4	4	4	4	4	4	4	4
120	3	3	3	3	3	3	3	3	3	
110	3	3	3	3	3	3	3	3		
100	2	2	2	2	2	2	2	2		
90	1	1	1	1	1	1	1	1		
80	1	1	1	1	1	1	1			
Wt.:	120	130	140	150	160	170	180	200	220	250+lbs.

ON TABLE II:

1. Find your age.
2. Opposite your age, locate your fitness index.
3. You will find your condition of Physical Fitness above your fitness-index number.

Table II
YOUR PHYSICAL FITNESS

Age	Excellent	Good	Fair	Poor
20	2	3	4	5
25	2	3	4	5
30	1	2	5	5
35	1	2	5	5
40	1	2	5	5
45	1	2	4	5
50	1	2	4	5
55	1	2	4	5
60	1	1	4	5
65+	1	1	4	5

*Author's modification of Physical Fitness Calculators, U.S. Dept. of Agriculture Forest Service, Equipt. Devel. Center, Missoula, Mont.

II. Women

START WITH TABLE I:

1. Find your body weight.
2. Locate your pulse rate in After-Exercise Pulse Rate column.
3. Opposite your pulse rate and above your age, find your fitness-index number.
4. Now go to Table II.

Table I
YOUR FITNESS-INDEX NUMBER

After-Exercise Pulse Rate									
180	5	5	5	5	5	5	5	5	5
170	5	5	5	5	5	5	5	5	5
160	5	5	5	5	5	5	5	5	5
150	5	5	5	5	5	5	5	5	5
140	5	5	4	4	4	4	4	4	4
130	4	4	3	3	3	3	3	3	3
120	4	3	3	3	3	3	3	3	3
110	3	3	3	3	3	3	3	3	3
100	3	2	2	2					
90	1	1	1	1					
80	1	1	1	1					
Wt.:	100	110	120	130	140	150	160	170	180	200+ lbs.

ON TABLE II:

1. Find your age.
2. Opposite your age, locate your fitness-index number.
3. You will find your condition of Physical Fitness above your fitness-index number.

Table II
YOUR PHYSICAL FITNESS

Age	Excellent	Good	Fair	Poor
20	3	4	5	5
25	3	4	5	5
30	2	4	4	5
35	2	4	4	5
40	2	3	4	5
45	1	3	4	5
50	1	2	4	5
55	1	2	4	5
60	1	2	4	5
65+	1	2	4	5

4. THE NUMBER OF CALORIES IN ALCOHOLIC BEVERAGES

$0.8 \times$ proof $\times$ ounces $=$ calories

Add 100 calories per drink for all sweetened alcoholic beverages.

Add 150 calories per drink for all sweetened alcoholic beverages that contain a milk product.

ALCOHOL IS KETOGENIC.

Two highballs or cocktails before dinner can amount to as much as one-fourth of your total daily calorie needs.

5. THE SALT CONTENT OF NATURAL FOODS

Here is a small sampling of commonly eaten foods; if listed as cooked, there is no added salt. Note that all fresh fruits are very low in sodium content. Amounts of sodium are expressed in milligrams (mg.). One level teaspoon of salt is 4 grams or 4,000 milligrams.

Apples, 1 medium; 1 mg.
Apricots, 2–3 medium; 1 mg.
Asparagus, 2/3 cup, cooked; 2 mg.
Bananas, 1 medium; 1 mg.
Beans, lima, 3½ oz., cooked; 2 mg.
Beans, snap, 1 cup, cooked; 2 mg.
Beef, roast, lean, 2 medium slices; 65 mg.
Beets, ½ cup, cooked, drained; 36 mg.
Blueberries, 1 cup; 1 mg.
Bluefish, 3½ oz., raw; 74 mg.
Broccoli, cooked, 2/3 cup; 10 mg.
Carp, 1 medium serving; 50 mg.
Cashew nuts, 4–5; 2 mg.
Catfish, 3½ oz., raw; 60 mg.
Clams, 4 large, soft; 40 mg.
Chicken, 1 medium serving; 50 mg.
Corn, 1 medium ear, cooked; 0.7 mg.
Cream, 1 tbsp.; 6 mg.
Half and half, 1 tbsp.; 14 mg.
Eggs, 1 medium; 66 mg.
Grapefruit, 1 large; 1 mg.
Grapes, 1 large bunch; 0.5 mg.
Ham, butt, fresh, 1 large slice, cooked; 70 mg.
Herring, 3½ oz., raw; 74 mg.
Kidney beans, 2/5 cup, cooked; 3 mg.
Lamb, lean, 3½ oz., cooked, sliced; 75 mg.
Lettuce, 3¼ oz., plain. 9 mg.
Milk (homogenized, low-fat, nonfat: similar sodium content), 50 mg.; buttermilk higher
Mushrooms, 10 small, raw; 15 mg.
Oatmeal, 1 cup, cooked; 0.8 mg.
Onions, 1 medium raw; 10 mg.
Oranges, 1 medium; 2 mg.
Peanuts, 20 nuts, roasted, not salted; 0.4 mg.
Pears, 1 medium, raw; 2 mg.
Peas, 3½ oz., cooked; 1.5 mg.
Pork, lean, roasted, medium portion; 70 mg.
Potatoes, 1 white, medium, raw; 3 mg.
Pumpkin, raw, 3½ oz.; 1 mg.

Tomato, 1 medium raw; 3 mg.
Tuna, raw, 3½ oz.; 37 mg.
Wheat, 1 cup sifted (white and whole wheat similar); 3 mg.

6. THE SALT CONTENT OF POPULAR PROCESSED AND PREPARED FOODS

Here is a list of some commonly used processed foods. The sodium content of these foods is either entirely or partly under the control of the manufacturer—samples for analysis were taken from ordinary market sources. Other foods not mentioned specifically in the same categories, for example, baby food, soups, TV dinners, contain comparable amounts of sodium.

Asparagus, canned, 4 oz., 271 mg.
Baby food, beef and egg noodle, 1 jar; 367 mg.
Baby food, oatmeal, 1 jar or 6 tbsp., dry; 134 mg.
Baby food, potato, 482 mg.
Baby food, vegetable with chicken, 1 jar; 320 mg.
Bacon, canned, 2 slices; 540 mg.
Beans, snap, 1 cup, solids and liquid; 550 mg.
Beef pot pie, 4½ in. diam.; 300 mg.
Beets, canned, ½ cup, drained; 196 mg.
Biscuit mix, ¼ lb.; 1,300 mg.
Bologna, 1 slice; 390 mg.
Bran flakes, 40%, ¾ cup; 340 mg.
Bread, 1 average slice; 120 mg.
Cake, 1/6 wedge of 9″ diam.; 200–400 mg.
Cheese, American, 1 oz.; 200 mg.
Cheese, processed, 1 oz.; 320 mg.
Cheese spread, 1 oz.; 455 mg.
Cheese straws, 3½ oz.; 721 mg.
Chocolate fudge topping, 1 oz.; 115 mg.
Cod, dried, lightly salted; 8,100 mg.
Corned beef, cooked, 3 slices; 803 mg.
Cornflakes, 1 cup; 165 mg.
Crab, canned, ½ cup; 850 mg.
Cream substitute, 1 tsp.; 17 mg.
Doughnut, average size, plain; 160 mg.
Frankfurter, 1 average size; 550 mg.
Gelatin dessert powder, 1 regular standard 3 oz. package; 288 mg.
Macaroni and cheese, canned, 3½ oz.; 304 mg.
Margarine, 1 pat; 100 mg.
Metrecal, 8 oz.; 225 mg.
Mushrooms, canned, ½ cup solids and liquid; 400 mg.
Noodles, plain, dry, 1 cup; 3 mg.
Olives, green, 3½ oz.; 2,400 mg.
Pancake and waffle mix, 3½ oz., dry; 1,433 mg.
Peanut butter, 1 tbsp.; 24 mg.
Peas, canned, drained, 3½ oz.; 236 mg.
Pie, apple, 1/6 wedge of 9″ diam.; 482 mg.

Pizza, average slice; 702 mg.

Popcorn, 8 oz., popped, with oil and salt; 349 mg.

Pickle, 1 large, dill; 1,428 mg.

Potato chips, 3 oz.; 1,000–1,500 mg.

Pretzel, 1 standard, 3 ring; 60 mg.

Rice Krispies, 1 cup; 280 mg.

Salad dressing, 1 tbsp.; 100–300 mg.

Soups

  Bouillion cube, 1, meat extract; 424 mg.

  Bouillion cube, 1, vegetable extract; 245 mg.

  Canned soups, all contain 3 servings per can:

    Beef Broth; 784 mg.

    Beef Broth with noodles; 645 mg.

    Beef with vegetables; 766 mg.

    Black bean; 934 mg.

    Celery; 904 mg.

    Creamed chicken; 804 mg.

    Chicken gumbo; 945 mg.

    Tomato; 915 mg.

Dry packaged soups contain the same large amounts of salt as canned soups.

Soy sauce, 1 tbsp.; 1,200 mg.

Tomato juice, canned, 3¼ oz.; 200 mg.

Treet, 2 oz.; 780 mg.

Tuna, canned, in oil, ¾ cup, solid and liquid; 800 mg.

7. FOODS HIGH IN POTASSIUM

Amounts of potassium are given in milligrams (mg.).

Asparagus, 2/3 cup, cooked; 278 mg.
Bananas, 1 medium; 370 mg.
Beans, lima; 1/3 cup, raw; 650 mg.
Beans, kidney, 2/5 cup, cooked; 340 mg.
Broccoli, cooked, 2/3 cup; 382 mg.
Corn, 1 medium ear, cooked; 280 mg.
Grapes, 1 large bunch; 200 mg.
Lettuce, 3½ oz., plain; 264 mg.
Molasses, blackstrap, 1 tablespoon; 957 mg.
Mushrooms, 10 small, raw; 414 mg.
Orange, 1 medium; 300 mg.
Peas, 3½ oz., cooked; 316 mg.
Potatoes, white, 1 medium, raw; 407 mg.
Pumpkin, raw, 3½ oz.; 340 mg.
Tomato, 1 medium, raw; 244 mg.

8. LOW-DENSITY PROTEIN FOODS OF PLANT ORIGIN*

Metric system equivalent estimator: 1 tablespoon = ½ ounce = 15 grams.

Vegetable	Calories in a 3½-Ounce Portion	Protein (in grams) in a 3½-Ounce Portion
Artichoke, 1 large	44	2.8
Asparagus	20	2.2
Bamboo shoots	27	2.6
Beans, dry white	340	22.3
dry red	343	22.5
dry calico	349	23
lima, green, raw	123	8.4
lima, dry	345	20.4
mung, dry	340	24.2
mung, sprouts	35	3.8
snap, green raw	32	1.9
snap, yellow, raw	27	1.7
soy, raw immature	134	11
soy, raw mature, dry	403	34
soy, dry mature, cooked	130	11
soy sprouts, raw	46	6.2
Beet greens, cooked	24	2.2
Beets, raw	43	1.6
Broccoli	30	3.2
Brussels sprouts	45	4.5
Cabbage	24	1.3
Cauliflower	27	2.7
Chard	25	2.4
Chervil	57	3.4
Chickpeas, dry	360	20.5
Collard greens	40	3.5
Corn, 1 medium ear	100	3.5
Cow peas, dry	343	22.8
Dandelion greens	45	2.7
Dock or sorrel	28	2.1
Eggplant	25	1.2
Endive	20	1.7
Escarole	20	1.7
Fennel	28	2.8
Indian spinach	19	1.8
Kale	38	4.2
Kohlrabi	29	2.0

*Showing the amount of protein in an average portion (3½ ounces).

Lamb's-quarters (pigweed)	43	4.2
Leeks	52	2.2
Lentils, dry	340	24.7
Lettuce, butterhead	14	1.2
iceberg	14	1.2
romaine	18	1.3
Mushrooms	28	2.7
Mustard greens	31	3.0
New Zealand spinach	19	2.2
Okra, 8–9 medium pods	36	2.4
Onion, 1 medium	36	1.2
Parsley	44	3.6
Peas, dry, mature	340	24.1
Peas, raw, mature	84	6.3
Peanuts, raw	543	25.5
Potato, raw, sweet	114	1.7
Potato, raw, white	76	2.1
Pumpkin	26	1.0
Squash, summer	19	1.1
winter	50	1.4
Turnip greens	28	3.0
Yam	101	2.0

Grains

Barley, dry	348	9
Bran	244	12.9
Corn grits	344	8.7
Millet	327	9.9
Oatmeal, dry	390	15
Peanut flour, defatted	371	47.9
Rice bran	276	13.3
Rice, brown	400	8
Rice, white	340	7
Rye flour, dark	327	16.3
Soy flour, full fat	405	6.7
Wheat, red bulgar	300	13
Wheat flour, all purpose	400	11.5
Wheat germ	360	27
Whole-wheat flour	333	13.3
Wild rice	300	11.5

Fruits

Banana, 1 small	85	1.1
Orange, 1 large	50	1.0
Pokeberry	23	2.6
Watermelon	26	0.5

Seeds

Pumpkin and squash seeds	553	29
Safflower seeds	615	19
Sunflower seeds	560	24

9. PROTEIN FOODS IN PORTIONS THAT CONTAIN SEVEN GRAMS OF PROTEIN

A. Low-Density Foods* (cooked unless stated)	Portion Weight and/or Size (practical approximations)	Calories
Asparagus	10 oz.	60
Bamboo shoots	10 oz.	60
Barley	2⅔ oz.	210
Bean sprouts (mung bean, type becoming popular in U.S.)	6¼ oz.	70
Beets, carrots, onions, leeks	11½ oz.	140
Broad-beans	1 oz.	100
Broccoli	7 oz.	65
Brussels sprouts	6 oz.	90
Cabbage	20 oz.	120
Calico beans	1 oz.	100
Cauliflower	9 oz.	60
Collard greens	5 oz.	70
Corn, fresh	7 oz.	170
Corn grits, dry	2¾ oz.	290
Dandelion greens	9 oz.	100
Egg white, one	1 tbsp.	28
Fava beans	3½ oz.	100
Fennel	6½ oz.	80
Garden cress (watercress)	9 oz.	85
Kale	6 oz.	80
Kohlrabi	12 oz.	100
Lentils	1 oz.	100
Lettuce (very tasty cooked in vegetable mixtures)	20 oz.	90
Lima beans (raw or cooked, dry)	3½ oz.	125
Lotus root	6 oz.	100
Mushrooms	8 oz.	70
Mustard greens	8 oz.	70
Nonfat milk products† dry powder (dry measure)	1¾ oz.	72
liquid	7 oz.	75
Okra	9 oz.	90
Parsley	7 oz.	90
Potato, white	6¼ oz.	165

*Remember that dry beans, legumes, and grains all increase by three times in quantity-volume after cooking, from water absorption. There is no practical alteration in food energy or protein content.
†Home-made yogurt or cottage cheese made from nonfat milk can be calculated from original amounts and estimated for losses in preparation.

Pumpkin, rutabaga, squash, turnip	21½ oz.	200
Rice (average of usual varieties), raw	3½ oz.	350
Soybeans (raw or cooked, dry)	1¾ oz.	125
Soybean products		
soybean curd	3½ oz.	70
miso bean paste	4 oz.	170
fermented soy beans	4 oz.	150
Snap beans	10 oz.	90
Spinach	6 oz.	40
Taro leaves and stems	6 oz.	100
Wheat (average of usual varieties)	1¾ oz.	150
Wheat flours (average)	2¾ oz.	300
Yam	9 oz.	300

B. Medium-Density Foods
Includes commercial preparations of low-fat cheese; read labels; 1 slice provides 7 grams of protein.

Codfish, mackerel, etc.	1 slice (2″ × 2″ × 1″)	75
Oysters, shrimp, clams	5 small	75
Salmon, tuna, crab (water-packed)	¼ cup	75
Sardines (water-packed)	3 medium	75

C. High-Density Foods

Cheese, cheddar, American	1 slice (3½″ × 1½″ × ¼″)	75
Cheese, cottage, uncreamed	¼ cup	75
Egg, whole	1	75
Meat and Poultry (beef, lamb, pork,		
liver, chicken, etc.—medium fat)	1 slice (4″ sq., ¼″ thick)	75
Cold cuts	1 slice (4½″ sq., ⅛″ thick)	75
Frankfurter	1 (8–9/lb.)	75
Milk		
whole milk	0.6 cup	100
evaporated milk	0.3 cup	100
buttermilk	0.6 cup	100
powdered whole milk	1½ tbsp.	100

D. Very High Density Food

Peanut butter	2 tbsp.	160
(10 gm. fat to 7 gm. protein)		

10. FIBER CONTENT OF FOODS

Fiber content is given in grams for a typical 3½-ounce portion.

Food (100 grams—3½ ounces—or as stated)	Fiber (grams)
Apple	1.0
Apricot, raw	0.6
Artichoke, cooked	2.4
Avocado	1.6
Banana	0.5
Beans: snap, lima, dry white, or red; dry, cooked	1.5
Bean sprouts, raw or cooked	0.7
Beet greens, cooked	1.1
Blackberries, raw	4.1
Blueberries, raw	1.5
Bran flakes, 40%, ¾ cup weighs 28 gm.	1.0
All-bran, ½ cup weighs 28 gm.	2.3
Bran, wheat, 1 tbsp.	1.0
Bran muffin	0.6
Bread, average for 1 slice of all white breads and rye	negligible
Bread, average for 1 slice whole-wheat types	0.3
Broccoli, cooked or raw	1.5
Cabbage, raw or cooked	0.8
Carrot, raw or cooked	1.0
Celery, raw or cooked	0.6
Corn, cooked	0.7
Cornbread, 1 average serving	0.3
Dates, 10 medium pitted (note: 275 calories)	2.3
Figs, dried, 5 medium (note: 275 calories)	5.6
Grapefruit	0.2
Grapes	0.6
Jicama (yambean), raw	0.7
Lentils, cooked	1.2
Lettuce	0.5
Mushrooms, canned or fresh	0.8
Mustard greens, cooked	1.0
Nuts, average portion of 1 oz.; cashews have ½ as much	0.7
Oatmeal, cooked, ¾ cup	0.4
Orange, raw, peeled	0.5

Orange juice	0.1
Papaya	0.9
Parsnip	2.0
Peaches, raw or canned	0.5
Peanuts, roasted with skin	2.7
Peanut butter, 1 tbsp.	0.9
Pears	1.4
Peas, green, cooked	2.0
Persimmon, raw	1.5
Pineapple	0.4
Plums, cooked or raw	0.4
Popcorn	2.2
Potato, baked, with skin	0.7
Prunes, dried, 8 large	2.0
Prune juice	negligible
Pumpkin, canned or fresh, cooked	1.3
Radishes, 1 oz.	0.2
Raspberries	3.0
Rhubarb, cooked	0.6
Rice, cooked, brown	0.3
Rice, cooked, white	0.1
Rice, puffed	0.6
Rice bran, 1 tbsp.	1.9
Sauerkraut	0.7
Seaweed, raw kelp	6.8
Irish moss	2.1
agar	0.7
Soybeans, cooked	1.7
Spinach, raw or cooked	0.6
Squash, summer, cooked	0.6
Squash, winter	1.8
Strawberries, raw	1.3
Sunflower seeds, 1 oz.	1.2
(pumpkin and squash seeds are slightly lower)	
Sweet potato, baked	0.9
Tomato, raw	0.5
Tomato juice	0.2
Turnip, cooked or raw	0.9
Turnip greens, cooked	0.7
Vegetables, mixed, frozen	1.2
Watercress, raw	0.7
Watermelon	0.3
Wheat, whole-grain, either unground,	
or cereal ground or fine; nothing removed	2.0
Wheat germ, 1 tbsp.	0.8

11. CARBOHYDRATE AND FAT FOODS CLASSIFIED ACCORDING TO DENSITY

A. Very Low-Density Vegetables

Vegetables listed are raw; you may eat as much as desired of raw vegetables.

Asparagus
Broccoli
Brussels sprouts
Cabbage
Carrots
Cauliflower
Celery
Chicory
Cucumbers
Eggplant
Escarole
Greens: beet, chard, collard,
   dandelion, kale, mustard,
   spinach, turnip

Lettuce
Mushrooms
Okra
Pepper, green or red
Radishes
Sauerkraut
String beans
Summer squash
Tomatoes
Turnips
Watercress

B. Low-Density Vegetables

Vegetables listed are cooked; each portion supplies approximately 7 grams of carbohydrate and 2 grams of protein, or 36 calories; 1 portion is ½ cup.

Beets
Carrots
Onions
Peas, green

Pumpkin
Rutabaga
Squash, winter
Turnips

C. Low-Density Fruits

Fruits—fresh, dried, or canned without sugar; each portion supplies approximately 10 grams of carbohydrate, approximately 40 calories.*

	Household Measurement
Apple	1 small (2″ diam.)
Applesauce	½ cup
*Apricots, fresh	2 medium
*Berries, black, boysen	1 cup
Blueberries	⅔ cup
Cantaloupe	¼ (6″ diam.)
Cherries	10 large
*Figs, fresh	2 large
Grapefruit	½ small

Grapefruit juice	½ cup
*Grapes	12
Grape juice	¼ cup
Honeydew melon	⅛ (7″)
Mango	½ small
*Orange	1 small
Orange juice	½ cup
Papaya	⅓
Peach	1 medium
Pear	1 small
Pineapple	½ cup
Pineapple juice	⅓ cup
Plums	2 medium
Tangerine	1 large
*Watermelon	1 cup

D. Medium-Density Fruits

Each portion supplies approximately 10 grams of carbohydrate, or 40 calories.

	Household Measurement
Apricots, dried	4 halves
Banana	½ small
Dates	2 small
Prunes, dried	2 small
Raisins	1½ tbsp.

E. Other Medium-Density Carbohydrate Foods

Each portion supplies approximately 15 grams of carbohydrate and 2 grams of protein, or approximately 68 calories.

	Household Measurement
Bread	1 slice
Biscuit, roll	1 (2″ diam.)
Muffin	1 (2″ diam.)
Cornbread	1½″ cube
Flour	2½ tbsp.
Cereal, cooked	½ cup
(flakes or puffed)	¾ cup
Rice or grits, cooked	½ cup
Spaghetti, noodles, etc.	½ cup

*These fruits contain about 1 gram of protein in the amounts listed. The figure of 40 calories is an approximation, because exact carbohydrate, protein, water, and fiber content vary with many factors, including soil, season, variety, etc.

Crackers, graham	2
oyster	20 (½ cup)
round	6–8
saltine	5
soda	3

F. High-Density Carbohydrate Foods

All human-made jams, jellies, preserves, pies, cakes, cookies, confections, sweetened rolls, icings, frostings, commercial gelatin desserts unless made with artificial sweetener, sugar- and honey-coated cereals, ice cream, and other fat and refined-sugar mixtures, and alcoholic beverages. A relatively small quantity of any of these foods contains large amounts of calories of food energy. For example, one inch-square brownie with nuts gives 200 calories; one average slice of Boston cream pie gives 500 calories, which is almost one-half of the total daily intake of 1,200 calories.

G. Fats and Oils: Always High-Density

Diet margarine contains more water than ordinary margarine; margarine is all human-made, thus cannot be "natural." Sour-cream substitutes require label reading for nutrient guidance. Each portion supplies approximately 5 grams of fat, or 45 calories (add 15–20 calories for sugar to cream-filled chocolate).

	Household Measurement
Avocado	⅛ (4″ diam.)
Butter or margarine	1 tsp.
Bacon, crisp	1 slice
Chocolate	1 miniature, cream-filled
Cream, light	2 tbsp.
Cream, heavy	1 tbsp.
Cream substitute, the same as cream, light	
Cream, sour	30 grams; 1 oz.
Cream cheese	1 tbsp.
French dressing	1 tbsp.
Mayonnaise	1 tsp.
Nuts	6 small
Oil or cooking fat	1 tsp.
Olives	5 small
Sauce, Hollandaise	1 tbsp. (scant)

12. HIGH-CALCIUM FOODS*

Food	Amount	Calcium (in milligrams)
Bok choy (or pak choy, uncurled, green cabbage)	3½ oz., cooked	165
Broccoli	3½ oz., cooked	100
Carob flour	3½ oz.	350
Cheese	1 oz.	150 to 325
Collard greens	3½ oz., cooked	200
Dandelion greens	3½ oz., cooked	190
Dried figs	5 medium	125
Kale	3½ oz., cooked	200
Milk (nonfat)	8 oz.	290
Molasses (blackstrap)	1 tbsp.	100
Mustard greens	3½ oz., cooked	200
Parsley	3½ oz., raw	200
Turnip greens	3½ oz., cooked	200
Watercress	3½ oz., raw	150
Yogurt (made with nonfat milk)	8 oz.	290

13. HIGH-PHOSPHORUS FOODS

Cheese
Dried beans
Egg yolk
Fish
Fowl
Grains

Highly processed foods
Meat
Milk
Seeds
Soda pop (highest phosphorus content of all foods)

*The average adult calcium requirement is only about 750 to 800 milligrams per day. The phosphorus requirement is the same. The problem is that many North Americans are getting too much phosphorus, which prevents calcium from being absorbed.

14. HIGH-IRON FOODS

Beans, white, red,
   calico, kidney,
   lima, mung,
   pinto
Beef
Blackeye peas
Buckwheat
Chard
Clams
Greens, dandelion,
   kale, mustard
Heart, beef, lamb,
   pork, turkey,
   chicken
Lentils
Lettuce

Millet
Oatmeal
Ocean perch
Parsley
Persimmon
Prunes, dry
Raisins
Rice bran
Rye, whole-grain
Sardines, canned
Seaweeds
Sesame seeds
Soybeans
Spinach
Watermelon
Yeast

15. FOODS HIGH IN VITAMINS A AND D

Vegetables

Beet greens
Broccoli
Carrots
Chicory
Collards
Cress
Dandelion greens
Escarole
Fennel
Kale
Lettuce

Mustard greens
Parsley
Pimento
Pumpkin
Spinach
Swiss chard
Sweet potato
Tamala leaves, raw
Turnip greens
Watercress
Winter squash

Milk products

All in United States and Canada are Vitamin A and D fortified; read labels for added amounts

Meat, Fish, Fowl

Eel
Eggs
Liver, all meats, fish and
   fowl

Lobster
Oysters
Swordfish
Whitefish

Fruits

Amaranth
Apricot
Cantaloupe
Cherries
Loquat
Mango

Mulberries
Nectarine
Papaya
Peach
Pokeberry

Grains, Cereals, Flours

Yellow corn, grits, mash, flour, popcorn

16. FOODS HIGH IN B VITAMINS

Foods High in Vitamin B₁ and Riboflavin

Vegetables

Asparagus
Beans, calico, dry
    kidney, dry
    lima, dry
    mung, dry
    soy, mature, raw

white, common, dry
Lentils
Mushrooms
Peanuts
Peas, fresh, dry and frozen

Fruits

Oranges
Prunes

Milk Products

All contain some, highest in evaporated milk and fresh whole milk

Meat, Fish, Fowl

Beef, organs
Ham
Liver, all meats and
    poultry
Lobster
Oysters
Pike

Pompano
Pork, all cuts
Roe, cod, herring, shad
Salmon
Spanish mackerel
Sturgeon
Turbot

Grains, Cereals, and Flours

Buckwheat flour
Bran, rice
Corn, yellow grits, flour,
    mash, popcorn
Oatmeal
Peanut flour

Rice flour, from unpolished
    rice
Soy flour
Wheat germ
Whole-wheat flour

Foods High in Niacin (Nicotinic Acid)

Vegetables

Artichoke
Asparagus
Beans, kidney, dry
Calico, dry
Corn

Lentils
Limas, dry and fresh
Lotus root
Mung beans, raw
Mushrooms

Peas, raw, dry, or frozen,   Peanuts
   chickpeas (garbanzos),   Potato
   cow peas

Grains, Cereals, Flours

Corn, all yellow-corn products, grits, mash, flour
Bran, wheat and rice
Peanut flour
Rye flour
Soy flour
Whole-wheat flour

Meat, Fish, and Fowl

Bass   Lobster
Beef, meat and organs   Mullet
Butterfish   Oysters
Cod   Porgy
Croaker   Salmon
Haddock   Shad
Heart, from all meats and   Swordfish
   fowl   Trout
Lamb   Tuna, fresh, canned
Liver

17. FOODS HIGH IN VITAMINS C, E, AND K

Vitamin C

Fruits

Acerola	Guava
Apricot	Honeydew
Blackberries	Kumquat
Cantaloupe	Lemon
Cherries	Lime
Currants, raw	Orange
Elderberries	Papaya
Gooseberries	Strawberries
Grapefruit	

Vegetables

Beans, snap, green and yellow, wax, sprouts, mung and soy	Mustard greens
Broccoli	Onions
Brussels sprouts	Parsley
Burdock	Peas, raw, green (approx. ½ vitamin C lost in freezing)
Cabbage, white, red, savoy	Pepper, green
Cauliflower	Pimentos
Chard	Potato (gradual loss between third and twelfth month of storage; no loss in baking)
Chayote	
Collard greens	
Cress	Rutabaga
Dandelion greens	Soybeans, immature, fresh
Dock (also called sorrel)	Spinach
Fennel	Sweet potato
Kale	Tampala greens
Kohlrabi	Turnip greens and root
Lamb's-quarters	

Vitamin E

All whole grains, seeds, beans, and legumes are high in Vitamin E

Vitamin K

All leafy vegetables

18. FOODS THAT CONTAIN RELATIVELY LARGE AMOUNTS OF EXOGENOUS CHOLESTEROL*

Food	Cholesterol (in milligrams per 100 grams or 3½ ounces)
Beef, raw, average cut	70
Brains, beef, raw	2,000
Butter	250
Caviar, or fish roe	300
Cheese, hard	120
cottage, creamed	15
low-fat: 25–30% fat	85
cream	100
Chicken, no skin, raw	60
Crabmeat	125
Egg, whole	550
Egg yolk	1,500
Fish, fillet or steak	70
Heart, raw	150
Lamb, raw	70
Liver, beef, raw	300
Ice cream	45
Margarine—⅔ animal fat and ⅓ vegetable fat (all vegetable oils have no exogenous cholesterol)	65
Milk, whole	11
whole dried	85
nonfat	3
Oysters	200
Pork	70
Shrimp	125
Sweetbreads	250
Veal	90

*Cholesterol made outside of the body.

19. RATIO OF POLYUNSATURATES TO SATURATES IN POPULAR FATTY FOODS

Group 1. High in polyunsaturates—ratio more than 2.5

Almonds	Imitation mayonnaise
Corn oil	Safflower oil
Cottonseed oil	Sesame oil
Mayonnaise	Soybean oil

Group 2. Polyunsaturates/saturates between 1.5 and 2.5

Chicken breast, skin, thigh
Fish, freshwater
Peanut oil

Group 3. Polyunsaturates/saturates between 0.5 and 1.5

Beef, heart, liver	etable oils
Chicken heart	Peanut butter
Fish, saltwater	Pecans
Hydrogenated (hardened) veg-	

Group 4. Polyunsaturates/saturates between 0.1 and 0.5

Chicken liver	Olive oil
Lard	Pork, all cuts

Group 5. Polyunsaturates/saturates less than 0.1

Beef, meat and fat	Milk and milk products, ex-
Butter	cept nonfat
Coconut oil	Mutton, fat and meat
Egg yolk	

20. FOODS HIGH IN INVISIBLE FAT

Each portion supplies approximately 5 grams of fat and 45 fat calories.

Food	Household Measurement
Avocado	⅛ (4″ diam.)
Butter or margarine	1 tsp.
Bacon, crisp	1 slice
Cream, light	2 tbsp.
Cream, heavy	1 tbsp.
Cream, substitute, dried	5 tsp.
Cream cheese	1 tbsp.
French dressing	1 tbsp.
Mayonnaise	1 tsp.
Mayonnaise, imitation	1 tbsp.
Nuts	
Almonds	9 nuts
Brazil nuts	2 medium
Butternuts	2 nuts
Cashews	4 nuts
Coconut, dried, shredded	1½ tbsp.
Filberts or hazel nuts	5–6 nuts
Hickory nuts	5 halves
Macadamia nuts	1¾ nuts
Mixed nuts, shelled	5–6 nuts
Pecans, shelled, halved	5 halves
Pine nuts	1 tbsp.
Walnuts, black	5–8 halves
Walnuts, English	4–7 halves
Olives	5 small

21. THE ORIGINAL EXCHANGE DIET AND HOW TO USE IT

List 1   Allowed as Desired
(need not be measured)

Seasonings: Cinnamon, celery salt, garlic, garlic salt, lemon, mustard, mint, nutmeg, parsley, pepper, saccharin and other sugarless sweeteners, spices, vanilla, and vinegar.

Other Foods: Coffee or tea (without sugar or cream), fat-free broth, bouillon, unflavored gelatin, rennet tablets, sour or dill pickles, cranberries (without sugar), rhubarb (without sugar).

Vegetables: Group A—insignificant carbohydrate or calories. You may eat as much as desired of raw vegetable. If cooked vegetable is eaten, limit amount to 1 cup.

Asparagus	spinach, turnip
Broccoli	Lettuce
Brussels sprouts	Mushrooms
Cabbage	Okra
Cauliflower	Peppers, green or red
Celery	Radishes
Chicory	Sauerkraut
Cucumbers	String beans
Eggplant	Summer squash
Escarole	Tomatoes
Greens: beet, chard, collard,	Watercress
dandelion, kale, mustard,	

List 2   Vegetable Exchanges

Each portion supplies approximately 7 grams of carbohydrate and 2 grams of protein, or 36 calories.

Vegetables: Group B—One serving equals ½ cup, or 100 grams.

Beets	Pumpkin
Carrots	Rutabagas
Onions	Squash, winter
Peas, green	Turnips

List 3   Fruit Exchanges
(fresh, dried, or canned without sugar)

Each portion supplies approximately 10 grams of carbohydrate, or 40 calories.

Fruit (cont.)

	Household Measurement	Weight of Portion
Apple	1 small (2″ diam.)	80 gm.
Applesauce	½ cup	100 gm.
Apricots, fresh	2 medium	100 gm.
Apricots, dried	4 halves	20 gm.
Banana	½ small	50 gm.
Berries	1 cup	150 gm.
Blueberries	2/3 cup	100 gm.
Cantaloupe	¼ (6″ diam.)	200 gm.
Cherries	10 large	75 gm.
Dates	2	15 gm.
Figs, fresh	2 large	50 gm.
Figs, dried	1 small	15 gm.
Grapefruit	½ small	125 gm.
Grapefruit juice	½ cup	100 gm.
Grapes	12	75 gm.
Grape juice	¼ cup	60 gm.
Honeydew melon	⅛ (7″)	150 gm.
Mango	½ small	70 gm.
Orange	1 small	100 gm.
Orange juice	½ cup	100 gm.
Papaya	1/3 medium	100 gm.
Peach	1 medium	100 gm.
Pear	1 small	100 gm.
Pineapple	½ cup	80 gm.
Pineapple juice	1/3 cup	80 gm.
Plums	2 medium	100 gm.
Prunes, dried	2	25 gm.
Raisins	2 tbsp.	15 gm.
Tangerine	1 large	100 gm.
Watermelon	1 cup	175 gm.

List 4   Bread Exchanges

Each portion supplies approximately 15 grams of carbohydrate and 2 grams of protein, or 68 calories.

	Household Measurement	Weight of Portion
Bread	1 slice	25 gm.
Biscuit, roll	1 (2″ diam.)	35 gm.
Cornbread	1½″ cube	35 gm.
Muffin	1 (2″ diam.)	35 gm.

Flour	2½ tbsp.	20 gm.
Cereal, cooked	½ cup	100 gm.
Cereal, dry		
(flakes or puffed)	¾ cup	20 gm.
Rice or grits, cooked	½ cup	100 gm.
Spaghetti, noodles, etc.	½ cup	100 gm.
Crackers, graham	2	20 gm.
Crackers, oyster	20 (½ cup)	20 gm.
Crackers, saltine	5	20 gm.
Crackers, soda	3	20 gm.
Crackers, round	6–8	20 gm.
Vegetables		
Beans (lima, navy, etc.), dry, cooked	½ cup	90 gm.
Peas (split peas, etc.), dry, cooked	½ cup	90 gm.
Baked beans, no pork	¼ cup	50 gm.
Corn	1/3 cup	80 gm.
Parsnips	2/3 cup	125 gm.
Potato, white, baked or boiled	1 (2″ diam.)	100 gm.
Potatoes, white, mashed	½ cup	100 gm.
Potatoes, sweet, or yams	¼ cup	50 gm.
Sponge cake, plain	1½″ cube	25 gm.
Ice cream		
(Omit 2 fat exchanges)	½ cup	70 gm.

List 5   Meat Exchanges

Each portion supplies approximately 7 grams of protein and 5 grams of fat, or 73 calories. (30 grams equal 1 ounce.)

	Household Measurement	Weight of Portion
Meat and poultry (beef, lamb, pork, liver, chicken, etc.) (med. fat)	1 slice (3″ × 2″ × ⅛″)	30 gm.
Cold cuts	1 slice (4½″ sq., ⅛″ thick)	45 gm.
Frankfurter	1 (8–9 per lb.)	50 gm.
Codfish, mackerel, etc.	1 slice (2″ × 2″ × 1″)	30 gm.
Salmon, tuna, crab	¼ cup	30 gm.
Oysters, shrimp, clams	5 small	45 gm.
Sardines	3 medium	30 gm.
Cheese, cheddar, American	1 slice (3½″ × 1½″ × ¼″)	30 gm.
Cheese, cottage	¼ cup	45 gm.

Egg	1	50 gm.
Peanut butter*	2 tbsp.	30 gm.

*Limit peanut butter to one exchange per day unless carbohydrate is allowed
 for in diet plan.

List 6   Fat Exchanges

Each portion supplies approximately 5 grams of fat, or 45 calories.

	Household Measurement	Weight of Portion
Avocado	⅛ (4″ diam.)	25 gm.
Bacon, crisp	1 slice	10 gm.
Butter or margarine	1 tsp.	5 gm.
Cream, light	2 tbsp.	30 gm.
Cream, heavy	1 tbsp.	15 gm.
Cream cheese	1 tbsp.	15 gm.
French dressing	1 tbsp.	15 gm.
Mayonnaise	1 tsp.	5 gm.
Nuts	6 small	10 gm.
Oil or cooking fat	1 tsp.	5 gm.
Olives	5 small	50 gm.

List 7   Milk Exchanges

Each portion supplies approximately 12 grams of carbohydrate, 8 grams of protein, and 10 grams of fat, or 170 calories.

	Household Measurement	Weight of Portion
Milk, whole	1 cup	240 gm.
Milk, evaporated	½ cup	120 gm.
*Milk, powdered	¼ cup	35 gm.
*Buttermilk	1 cup	240 gm.

*Add 2 fat exchanges if milk is fat-free.

How to Work Out Your Diet with the Original Exchange System

Look at the left-hand column of the table, find the calories of food energy you wish to eat, then eat the number of each food group called for by your calorie choice.

Calories	Milk	Vegetable A	Vegetable B	Fruits	Bread Exchange	Meat Exchange	Fat Exchange
1,200	1 pt.	as desired	1	3	4	5	1
1,500	1 pt.	" "	1	3	6	6	4
1,800	1 pt.	" "	1	3	8	7	5
2,200	1 pt.	" "	1	4	10	8	8
2,600	1 qt.	" "	1	4	12	7	11
2,600, less milk	1 pt.	" "	1	4	12	10	12
3,000	1 pt.	" "	1	4	15	10	15

NOTE: It is now being widely recognized that this arbitrary "balancing" led to diets that were too high in fat and often too high in protein for most overweight people.

THE BREAK THE RULES CALORIE COUNTER*

The portions shown contain approximately 200 calories, or about one-fifth to one-sixth of your total daily calorie requirement.

A

Alcoholic beverages, average approximations shown here. For the calorie count of a specific
  beverage, see page 192.
  Beer, 16 ounces
  Brandy, 1¾ to 2 ounces
  Champagne, 7½ ounces
  Liqueur, 1 2/3 to 2 ounces
  Wine, 8 2/3 ounces
Almonds, 20 to 25 whole nuts
Anchovies, 27 thin fillets
Apple cider, 14 ounces
Apple dumpling, ⅝ of a dumpling
Apple fritter, ¾ of a fritter
Apple sauce, lightly sweetened, 12 T
  unsweetened, 20 T
Apricots, dried, 2½ large halves
  canned, in heavy syrup, 16 T, solids and liquid
  light syrup, 24 T, solids and liquids
  nectar, 12 ounces
Avocado, 8 T, mixed with mayonnaise, 7 T

B

Bacon, thin slices, well cooked and drained, 6 pieces
Bacon, Canadian, thin slices, well cooked, 4 pieces
Baconettes, roasted pork rinds, well cooked, 2 2/3 T
Bagel, with 1 pat of butter or margarine, 1
Beans, baked with molasses sauce and pork, 7 T
Beans and frankfurters, 8¾ T
Beans and ground beef (same as chili con carne), 7 T
Beans, refried, 6 2/3 T
Beef, very lean, no bone, no gravy, 3″ × 2″ × ⅛″, 3 pieces
Beef, fat with lean, 3″ × 2″ × ⅛″, 1¾ pieces
Beef and noodles (macaroni, spaghetti, chili mac.), 14 T
Beef, chopped, 4½ T
Beef goulash, 13 T
Beef hash, 6 2/3 T
Beef pie, with crust, 3¾ T
Beef stew, 7 2/3 T
Beef stroganoff, 4 2/3 T
Biscuit, baking powder, 2 medium
  egg, regular or diet, 4 medium
  sugared, 3¾ medium
Blintzes, cheese, 2½ T
  fruit, 2¾ T

*Liquid portions are given in ounces. The portion for foods that are soft enough to press into
a spoon are given in tablespoons, abbreviated T. All other foods are given in terms of pieces
with measurements when indicated.

Bologna, all meat, 2 thin slices
   with cereal, 2½ thin slices
Braunsweiger, 2 thin slices
Bread, deduct ½ slice if small amount of butter, margarine, honey, jam, or jelly is used
   Boston brown, 2 thin slices
   cheese, cinnamon, raisin, corn, cracked wheat, egg, 2½ thin slices
   date-nut, panetone, 2 thin slices
   English muffin, 1½
   gingerbread, 2″ × 2″ × ¼″ piece
   Hollywood, 4 thin slices
   bread sticks, 20 small, 4 large
   popover, 1 1/3
Butter or margarine, 2 T, diet margarine, 3½ T
Burritos, 6 T

C

Cabbage rolls, 8 T or 2 small rolls, stuffed with meat, with gravy
Cake
   angel food, 3 2/3 T, 2″ × 2″ × 1″
   plain white, 3¾ T, 2″ × 2″ × 1″, with icing, 3 1/3 T
   caramel, butterscotch, other flavors, 3¼ T, 2″ × 2″ × ¾″, with icing, 3 T
   chocolate, 3 T, 1½″ × 1¼″ × 1″, with icing, 2 1/3 T
   cheese, 5 T, with cherries, pineapple, or other fruit, 2½ T
   jelly roll, 5 T
Candy
   apple, 1 medium
   chocolate, diet, 3–4 pieces
   chocolate fudge, 1½ pieces
   M & Ms,™ 2¾ T
   chocolate covered nuts, 2¼ T
      peanuts, 1¼ T
      raisins, 3½ T
      vanilla creams, 1½ pieces
   gum drops, 4 T
   hard candy, 3¾ T
   honeycombed candy, chocolate covered, 3½ T
   licorice, 4 T
   peanut brittle, 3½ T
Candied fruit, 4 T
Cashews, 16 large, 20 medium
Cheese
   hard (romano, parmesan), 2½ T
   medium (cheddar, Monterey jack, colby, muenster, Edam, Swiss, American, processed
      brick), 2½ slices, 3½″ × 1½″ × ¼″
   soft (camembert, leiderkranz, bel paese, cream), 4 T
Cheese fondue, 7 1/3 T
Cheese souffle, 6½ T
Cheese spread 2 2/3 T
Chicken, a la king, 12 T
   cacciatore, 12 T
   chopped liver, with chicken fat and mayonnaise, 4¾ T
   creamed, 7¼ T
   fried with breading, 1 medium size leg
   pie, 6 T, with crust, 5 T
   stew, 12 T

with dumplings, 8 T
with noodles, 8 T
Chocolate drink, with water, 14 ounces; with nonfat milk, 6½ ounces; with whole milk, 5¾ ounces
Cookies
brownie with nuts, ¼ piece of a 2″ square
butter, 6 small
chocolate covered, 2 small
chocolate chip, 1¾ small, with nuts, 1¼ small
fig bar, 1½ small
fruit bar, 3 small
ginger snap, 6
macaroon, 2 medium
marshmallow, 2 medium
oatmeal, 2 medium
peanut, 1½ small
plain vanilla, 8 small
sandwich, 2
shortbread, 4 small
sugar, 2½ medium
Coffee cake
apple crispy, 3½ T
bear claw, 7 T
butter horn, 3½ T
with nuts, butter, syrup or honey, 3 T
Cornbread, 6 T
spoonbread, 6 T
Corn fritter, 3¼ T
Corn souffle, 9¼ T
Crackers, arrowroot, 9
cheese, ¾″ × ¾″, 25 to 30
flavored, bacon, cheese, chicken, onion
small, 25 pieces
medium, 12 pieces
large, 5 pieces
Graham, 2½″ × 2½″, 6, honey flavored, 5
matzo, 1⅝ pieces, flavored, 1½ pieces
oyster, 16
pilot, 4½ pieces
saltines, 8 pieces
soda, 8 pieces
tortilla chips, 2″ × 1½″, 18 to 20 pieces
Cream, half and half, 20 T
sour, 7½ T, imitation, depends on composition, varies from 4 to 7½ T
heavy or light whipping, 4 T

D

Danish pastry, see coffee cake
Dates, 3½
Desserts, apple brown betty, 7 T
bread pudding, 7 T, with nuts, 5 T
gelatin dessert, 5 T, with fruit, 4¼ T
chocolate pudding, 8 T
charlotte russe with ladyfingers and whipped cream, 5 T
plum pudding, 4½ T

tapioca pudding, 12 T
vanilla pudding, blancmange, 11 T
Dip, average from mixes, 5¼ T
Donut, small, plain, 1½, iced, ¾
Duck, flesh only, 4 oz., with skin, 2 oz.

E

Eclair, ¾ of an eclair
Egg, fried in butter, 2 large
    omelet with milk, cooked in fat, 1¾ large eggs
Egg nog, 10 T, with alcohol, 2½ T
Egg roll, 7 T
Egg substitute, equivalent of 4 large eggs, 3 if fried in fat
Enchilada, with meat or cheese, 6 T, with chili gravy, 5 T

F

Figs, dried, 3½
Fish, breaded and fried, 4 oz.
    cake, fried, 4 oz.
    gefilte fish, 2 1/3 pieces
Frankfurter, all meat, 1 1/3, with cereal, 1¾
French toast, 2 slices, with butter/margarine and syrup, 1½ slices

G

Ginger, candied, 4 T
Goose, flesh only, 5 T, with skin, 3⅛ T
Granola, honey coated cereal, plain 12 T, with raisins and nuts, 10 T
Gravy, 7 T

H

Ham, canned, very lean, no gravy, 3″ × 2″ × ⅛″, 3 pieces
    deviled, 4 T
    smoked, same as canned
Hamburger, with relish on a bun, quarter pounder, ½ of total; with cheese, 1/3 of total; eighth
    pounder, 2/3 of total; with chili con carne (chili size), ½ of total
Headcheese, 2½ 1-ounce slices
Herring, in sauce, cream, tomato or wine, 2″ × 3″ × ½″, 2 pieces
Honey, 3¼ T
Hors d'oeuvres, candied pickles, 12 very small
    caramel coated popcorn with peanuts, 1 regular package, 1⅜ ounces
    cheese flavored popcorn, 3 cups
    cheese straws, 6½ pieces
    chips, bacon, corn, or potato, 18 to 20 pieces
    little franks, 4 pieces; franks in a blanket, 3 pieces
    liver pate, 4 T
    liver wrapped with bacon, 3 pieces
    smoked salmon (lox), 2″ × 3″ × ¼″, 4 pieces
Hot dog on a bun with relish, 2/3 of total

I

Ice cream, average fat content, hard or soft
    chocolate, 6 T
    diet, 7½ T

vanilla or fruit flavors, 7 T
with nuts added to any flavor, 5 T
with sauces and topping (sundae), 2½ T
Ice milk, 9 T
Ices, 15 T
Instant breakfast, see chocolate drink, other flavors are comparable

J

Jam or jelly, 3¾ T

K

Kielbasa, 4½T
Knockwurst, 3 oz.

L

Lamb, comparable to beef
Lard, 1¾ T
Lasagne, 14 T
Lemonade, see soft drinks
Liver, fried, 6 T
Lobster Newburg, 6 T
  salad, 12½ T
Lunch meat, ⅛" thick, 2 1/3 slices

M

Macaroni, with meat or cheese or both, comparable to beef and noodles
  salad, 9 T
Malted milk, comparable to chocolate drink made with milk
Manicotti, with sauce, 6½ T
Maple syrup, see syrup
Margarine, 2 T
  diet or imitation (made by whipping in equal part of water), 4 T
Marmalade, comparable to jam and jelly
Mayonnaise, 2 T
  diet or imitation, 4 T
Meat casserole, with meat, noodles, 14 T (if significant amount of vegetables and no fat is
  added, density is lowered so that up to twice as much can be eaten)
Meat loaf, 5½ T, canned main meal meat, 6 T
Mexican dinner, ¼ of a medium combination platter
Milk shake, all flavors, with nonfat milk, 10¼ ounces, with whole milk, 7½ ounces
Molasses, blackstrap, 4 T
Muffin, 3" diameter, 1¾, with butter or margarine, 1 1/3, with raisins, plain, 1½

N

Nuts, mixed, dry or oil roasted, 2½ T

O

Oil, including olive, 1 2/3 T
Olives, 25 to 30 medium

P

Pancakes, 4" thick, 2, with butter or margarine, honey, jam, or syrup, 1½
Pastrami, comparable to sliced beef

Pastry, see coffee cake
    strudel, 2″ × 2″ × ½″
    turnovers, all flavors, 2/3 of a turnover
Peanut butter, 2 T
Peanuts, shelled 2½ T
Pecans, 24 to 28 halves
Pickles, sweet, 10 small
Pie, Boston cream, scant 1/12 of an 8″ pie
    chocolate cream, scant 1/12 of an 8″ pie, banana cream, comparable
    fruit flavors, 1/12 of a 9″ pie, includes mince and raisin
    lemon chiffon, scant ⅛ of an 8″ pie, other chiffon flavors comparable
Pineapple, crushed with syrup, 15 T
Pine nuts (pignolias), 2½ T
Pizza, 6 T, with sausage, 5 T
Pop bar, twin, frozen fruit flavors, 3½ bars
Pork, roasted, lean and fat, 4 T, lean only, 5¾ T
Pork sausage, cooked (16 links per pound), 2 1/3 links
Pork, sweet and sour, 5 T
Potato, chips, 2″ diameter, 18 to 20
    French fries, 2″ × ½″ × ½″, 12
    hash browned, 6 T
    mashed with milk and butter, 8 T
    salad, with mayonnaise and hard cooked eggs, 10 T
    scalloped, 5¼ T
Prunes, dried, large, 10

R

Raisins, 6 T
Ravioli, chicken or meat, with sauce, 14 T
Relish (barbecue, hamburger, hot dog, piccalili, sweet and sour), 6 T
Rice, fried, 11 1/3 T, flavored rice mixes are comparable
    Spanish, 17 T

S

Salad dressing, average, 3 T, with cheese, 2¾ T, diet, 4 to 8 T, depends on contents
Salami, cooked, 2½ ounces
    dry, 1 1/3 ounces
Salisbury steak, with mushroom gravy, 4 oz.
Sandwich spread, 3 1/3 T
Sardines, packed in oil, 5 T, packed in water, 8 T
Sauce, barbecue, 6 T
    cheese, 4½ T
    cocktail, 6 T
    cranberry, 8 T
    hard, 2½ T
    Hollandaise, 4½ T
    Newburg, 8 T
    savory, 10 T
    seafood, 8 T
    soy, 16 T
    white, medium thickness, 8 T
Shake and Bake, chicken, fish, and meat coating, 4 T
Sherbet, all flavors, 10½ T
Shrimp, breaded and fried, tempura is comparable, 3 large or 4 medium shrimp
Shrimp roll, comparable to egg roll

Snacks, see crackers, hors d'oeuvres, potato chips

Soup, average, with vegetables, small amount of lean meat, fish or seafood, 15 T
  bisques, creamed soups, 7 T

Soft drinks, cool-ade types, carbonated (all flavors), fruit juice mixtures with sugar added, punch, 15 ounces, instant orange, grapefruit, or grape breakfast drink, 13 T

Spaghetti, see beef and noodles

Sugar, beet or cane, no difference in calories
  confectioners, 8 T
  granulated, 4 T
  lump, 8 pieces
  maple, 1¾ × 1½ × ½″, 2 pieces

Sunflower seeds, shelled, 3 T

Sweetbreads, cooked, 6 T

Sweet potato or yam, candied, 12 T

Sweet potato pie, 6 2/3 T

Syrup, 4 T
  diet, variable, consult labels

T

Taco, beef-filled, 1 large, or 4 cocktail-size

Tamale, 5½ T

Tea mix, 10 1/3 teaspoons, low calorie, 50 teaspoons

Toaster baked products, 1 piece

Tongue, comparable to beef, lamb, pork

Topping, butterscotch, caramel, chocolate or chocolate flavored, fruit or nut flavored, marshmallow, 3½ T
  whipped, average of brands, 13 T

Tuna and noodles, 16 T
  pie, 8 T
  salad, 8 T

Turkey, flesh only, 5 oz., flesh and skin, 4 oz.
  casserole, 8 T (turkey and noodles, tetrazini, comparable)
  pie, 7 T

V

Veal parmigiana, 5 oz.

Veal roast, 4 oz.

W

Waffle, 1, ½″ × 4½″ × 5½″, plain; with butter or margarine, honey, jam, jelly, or syrup, ½

Walnuts, chopped, 4 T, 16 to 28 halves

Welsh rarebit, 7 T

Y

Yogurt, sweetened and flavored, made from low-fat milk, 12½ T

BIBLIOGRAPHY

APPETITE, HUNGER, AND SATIETY

Grossman, M.I. Satiety Signals. Am. J. Clin. Nutrition, 8:565, 1960.
Hashim, S.A., and Van Itallie, T.B. Studies in Normal and Obese Subjects with a Monitored Food Dispensing Device. Annals N.Y. Acad. of Sciences, 131:654, Oct. 8, 1965.
Kennedy, G.C. The Role of Depot Fat in the Hypothalamic Control of Food Intake in the Rat. Proc. Royal Biol. Soc. London, 140:578, 1953.
Stunkard, Albert. Obesity and the Denial of Hunger. Psychosomatic Med., 21:281, 1959.
Stunkard, Albert. New Therapies for the Eating Disorders: Behavior Modification of Obesity and Anorexia Nervosa. Arch. Gen. Psychiat., 26:391, May 1972.

NIBBLING

Laveille, Gilbert A., and Romsos, Dale R. Meal Eating and Obesity. Nutrition Today, 9:4, Nov.-Dec. 1974.

OVERWEIGHT, INSULIN, AND DIABETES

Grey, N., and Kipnis, D.M. Effect of Diet Composition On the Hyperinsulinemia of Obesity. N. Engl. J. Med., 285:827, 1971.
Hearings Before the Select Committee on Nutrition and Human Needs of the United States Senate, 93rd Congress, 1st Session. Part 2, Sugar in Diet, Diabetes, and Heart Diseases and Part 3. Appendix to Hearings. (For sale by the U.S. Govt. Printing Office, Washington, D.C. 20402.)
Hill, F.W. Nutrition Society Symposium. Energy Costs of Intermediate Metabolism in Intact Animal. Fed. Proc., 30:1434, 1971.
Neel, James V. Diabetes Mellitus: A "Thrifty" Genotype Rendered Detrimental by "Progress"? Am. J. Human Genetics, 14:353, Dec. 1962.
West, Kelly M., and Kalbfleisch, John M. Influence of Nutritional Factors on Prevalence of Diabetes. Diabetes, 20:99, Feb. 1971.

FAT CELLS AND BROWN FAT

Dole, Vincent P. Body Fat. Scientific American, 201:71, Dec. 1959.
Nelson, Ralph A. Winter Sleep in the Black Bear, A Physiologic and Metabolic Marvel. Mayo Clin. Proc., 48:733, Oct. 1973.

WHAT ARE NORMAL LEVELS OF BLOOD CHOLESTEROL?

Wright, Irving S. Correct Levels of Serum Cholesterol, Average vs Normal vs Optimal. JAMA, 236:261, July 19, 1976.

OVERWEIGHT RAISES BLOOD FAT LEVELS

Nichols, Allen B., et al. Independence of Serum Lipid levels and Dietary Habits. JAMA, 236:1948, Oct. 25, 1976. (The final conclusion of this detailed public health study is "weight reduction should be the initial intervention for control of hyperlipidemia in the general population.)

SCIENTIFIC STUDY DEMONSTRATING HOW LOW-DENSITY EATING LEADS TO WEIGHT LOSS AND LOWER BLOOD FAT

Sacks, Frank, M., et al. Plasma Lipids and Lipoproteins in Vegetarians and Controls. New Engl. J. Med., 292:1148, May 29, 1975. (This study found that "The vegetarians, in addition to having lower lipid levels than the controls, weighed less and were leaner.")

BLOOD FAT LEVELS OF ESKIMOS

Bang, H.O., and Dyerberg, J. Plasma Lipids and Lipoproteins in Greenlandic West Coast Eskimos. Acta. Med. Scand., 192:85, 1972. (Recent reports indicate that as these people intermarry with non-Eskimos, and eat more saturated fat and sugar, the foods typical of the United States, they are succumbing more and more to diabetes and cholesterol diseases.)

PHYSICAL ACTIVITY

Mann, George V. Medical Progress: The Influence of Obesity on Health. New Engl. J. Med., 291:178 and 226, July 25 and Aug. 1, 1974. ("Physical inactivity may need to be considered the prime cause of several of industrial man's chronic diseases, including obesity.")

Marston, A.R., London, P., Lammas, S.E. Lifestyle: A Behavioral Program For Weight Reduction and Obesity Research. Bariatric Med., 5:376, May-June, 1976.

THE METABOLIC COST OF PHYSICAL ACTIVITY: CALORIES BURNED FROM WORK AND EXERCISE

The Approximate Metabolic Cost of Activities, prepared by the American Heart Association.

BODY HEAT LOSS AND THE INCREASE OF THIS LOSS FROM EXERCISE

Miller, D.S., Mumford, P., Stock, M.J. Gluttony: Thermogenesis in Overeating Man. Am. J. Clin. Nutr., 20:1223, 1967.

FACTORY WORKERS ATE MORE WHEN THEY WORKED LESS

Mayer, J. and Mitra, R.P. Relation Between Caloric Intake, Body Weight and Physical Work. Am. J. Clin. Nutr., 4:169, 1956.

HIGH PROTEIN DIETS

Banting, William. Letter on corpulence addressed to the Public. Ed. 2 London, Harrison, 1963.

Bazaar's New Nine-Day Wonder Diet. Harper's Bazaar, 107:19, July, 1974.

Cannon, Poppy. The Great Nova Scotia Diet. Ladies' Home Journal, 83:114, March 1966.

De Ville, M. The Digital Dieters' Handbook. Denville, N.J.: Hartford Pub. Corp., 1973.

Elting, L. Melvin, and Isenberg, Seymour. You Can Be Fat Free Forever. N.Y.: St. Martin's Press, 1974.

Fredericks, Carlton. Dr. Carlton Frederick's Low Carbohydrate Diet. N.Y.: Award Books, 1965.

Friedman, Abraham I. Fat Can Be Beautiful. N.Y.: Berkley, 1974.

Hauser, Gayelord. The New Diet Does It. N.Y.: Berkley, 1972.

Hayden, Naura. The Hip, High-Prote, Low-Cal, Easy-Does-It Cookbook. N.Y.: Dell, 1972.

Olympic Diet. Epicure, Summer, 1973.

Pennington, Alfred W. The Use of Fat in a Weight-Reducing Diet. Del. St. M.J. 23: 79, April, 1951.

Perlstein, Irving B., with Cole, William. Diet Is Not Enough. N.Y.: Collier-Macmillan Co., 1972.

Petrie, Sidney, and Stone, Robert B. The Lazy Lady's Easy Diet. West Nyack, N.Y.: Parker Pub. Co., 1969.
Petrie, Sidney, and Stone, Robert B. The Miracle Diet for Fast Weight Loss. West Nyack, N.Y., Parker Pub. Co., 1970.
Riccio, Otone and Dolores. The Weighing Game and How to Win It. Emmaus, Pa.: Rodale Press, 1974.
Salisbury, J.H. Brief Statement of the So-called Salisbury Plans. London, Balliere, 1887.
Stillman, Irwin M., and Baker, Samm S. The Doctor's Quick Weight Loss Diet. N.Y.: Dell, 1967.
Stillman, Irwin. M., and Baker, Samm S. Dr. Stillman's 14-Day Shape-Up Program. N.Y.: Delacorte Press, 1974.
The Wisconsin Diet. McCall's, 90:26, July 1963.

KETOSIS AND DAMAGE TO THE UNBORN CHILD

Adamsons, Karlis. Hearings Before the Select Committee on Nutrition and Human Needs of the United States Senate, 93rd Congress. Part 1-Obesity and Fad Diets. Washington, D.C., April 12, 1972. U.S. Government Printing Office, Washington, D.C., 1973.

KETOSIS AND CALCIUM REMOVAL FROM BONE

Avioli, Louis V. Report to Institute of Human Nutrition, College of Physicians and Surgeons of Columbia University, reviewed in Hospital Tribune, 10:2, Feb. 2, 1976.

THE HARVARD STUDY OF THE STILLMAN HIGH PROTEIN DIET:

Rickman, Frank, et al. Changes in Serum Cholesterol During the Stillman Diet. JAMA, 228:54, April 1, 1974.

HIGH FAT DIETS

Arai, Hirohisa. Eat and Become Slim—A Beauty Diet with Vegetable Oil. Tokyo: Shufunotomo Co., Ltd., 1972.
Atkins, Robert C. Dr. Atkins' Diet Revolution. N.Y.: David McKay, 1972. Articles criticizing Dr. Atkins' diet: Item 3-Articles Pertinent to Hearing Pertaining to Dr. Atkins' "Diet" pp. 61–78 of: Hearings Before the Select Committee on Nutrition and Human Needs of the United States Senate, 93rd Congress. Part I-Obesity and Fad Diets. Washington, D.C., April 12, 1972, U.S. Govt. Printing Office, Washington, 1973.
Berman, Sam S. The Boston Police Diet and Weight Control Program. N.Y.: Frederick Fell, 1972. Renunciation of The Boston Police Diet: Berland, T. Consumer's Guide: Rating The Diets. p. 283, Skokie, Ill.: Publications International, Ltd.
McMahon, Ed. Slimming Down. N.Y.: Grosset and Dunlap, 1972.
Mart, Donald S. The Carbo-Calorie Diet. Garden City, N.Y.: Doubleday and Co., 1973.
Pennington, Alfred W. Treatment of Obesity: Developments of the Past 150 Years. Am. J. Dig. Dis. 21:65, 1964.
Petrie, Sidney, and Stone, Robert. Fat Destroyer Foods: The Magic Metabolizer Diet. West Nyack, N.Y.: Parker Pub. Co., 1974.
Petrie, Sidney and Stone, Robert. Martinis and Whipped Cream. West Nyack, N.Y.: Parker Pub. Co., 1966.
Reinsh, Ernest R. Eat, Drink and Get Thin. N.Y.: Hart Pub. Co., 1969.
Taller, Herman. Calories Don't Count. N.Y.: Simon and Schuster, 1961.
Tarr, Yvonne Y. The New York Times Natural Foods Dieting Book. N.Y.: Quadrangle/The N.Y. Times Book Co., 1972.
Thorpe, George L. M.D. Gives Simple Diet for Fast Weight Loss. Sci. News Letter Nov. 30, 1957.
Wernick, Robert. I Wrote The Drinking Man's Diet. Sat. Eve. Post, May 22, 1965.
The Drinking Man's Danger. Time, March 5, 1965.
Yudkin, John, Ed. Sweet and Dangerous. N.Y.: Peter H. Wyden, Inc., 1972.

THE KETOGENIC AND HYPOGLYCEMIC PROPERTY OF ALCOHOL

Gastineau, Clifford F. Nutrition Note: Alcohol and Calories. Mayo Clinic Proceedings, 51:88, Feb. 1976.

FASTING AND MODIFIED FASTING

Blackburn, George L. Letter to The American Society of Bariatric Physicians: Newsletter, Am. Soc. of Bariatric Phys., April-May, 1976.

Cott, Allan. Fasting: The Ultimate Diet. N.Y.: Bantam Books, 1975.

Genuth, Saul, et al. Weight Reduction in Obesity by Outpatient Semistarvation. JAMA, 230:987, Nov. 18, 1974.

Linn, Robert. Dr. Linn's Last Chance Diet. Secaucus, N.J.: Lyle Stuart, 1976.

White, Philip L. At Last, The Ultimate Diet: Total Fasting (Total Foolishness). American Medical News, Jan. 19, 1976.

BACKGROUND ON FASTING

Alexander, Shana. The Zero Calorie Diet. Life, 55:105, Oct. 11, 1963.

Drenick, Ernst J., et al. Prolonged Starvation as Treatment for Severe Obesity. JAMA, 187:140, Jan. 11, 1964.

LOW CALORIE BALANCED DIETS

Antonetti, Vincent. The Computer Diet. N.Y.: M. Evans and Co., 1973.

Bennett, Iva, and Simon, Martha. The Prudent Diet. N.Y.: David White, 1973.

Berland, Theodore. Rating the Diets. (Dr. Smith's Astronaut's Diet, page 317.) Skokie, Ill.: Publications International, Ltd.

Cadence Computerized Diet. West Des Moines, Iowa.

Christakis, George. Wise Woman's Diet. Redbook, 128:37, 1967.

Dolger, Jonathan. The Expense Account Diet. N.Y.: Random House, 1969.

The Editor's Diet. Mademoiselle, 64:184, April, 1957.

Englehardt, S.L. The Workingman's Diet. The Reader's Digest, 100:53, Jan. 1972.

Evan, Frances. Ladies' Home Journal Family Diet Book. N.Y.: Macmillan, 1973.

Friedman, Abraham. How Sex Can Keep You Slim. Englewood Cliffs, N.J.: Prentice Hall, 1972.

Gage, Joan. The Amazing "New You" Diet. Ladies' Home Journal, 88:130, March, 1971.

Glenn, Morton B. But I Don't Eat That Much. N.Y.: Dutton, 1974.

Jolliffe, Norman. The Prudent Man's Diet. House Beautiful, 103:104, Jan. 1961.

Mayo Clinic Diet Manual. Philadelphia: W.B. Saunders Co., 1971.

Proxmire, William. You Can Do It! N.Y.: Simon and Schuster, 1973.

Shedd, Rev. Charlie W. The Fat Is in Your Head. Word, 1972.

Small, Marvin. The Easy 24 Hour Diet. Garden City, N.Y.: Doubleday and Co., 1973.

Solomon, Neil, and Knudson, Mary. Dr. Solomon's Easy, No-Risk Diet. N.Y.: Coward, McCann and Geoghegan, 1974.

Wyden, Peter, Overweight Society, N.Y.: Morrow, 1965.

HIGH FIBER DIETS

Fredericks, Carlton. The High Fiber Way to Health. N.Y.: Pocket Books, 1975.

Rubin, David. The Save Your Life Diet. N.Y.: Random House, 1975.

BACKGROUND ON HIGH FIBER DIETS

Burkitt, D.P., Walker, A.R.P., et al. Effect of Dietary Fiber. Lancet, 2:1408, 1972.

Connell, Alastair M. Dietary Fiber and Diverticular Disease. Hospital Practice. 12:119, March 1976.

CRASH DIETS CAUSING HAIR LOSS

Goette, Detlef F., and Odom, Richard B. Alopecia in Crash Dieters. JAMA 235:2622, June 14, 1976.

REGULATORY AGENCIES AND WEIGHT LOSS

Relaxacizor vs. FDA: FDA Consumer Memo: Relaxacizor. Current and Useful Information From The FDA. U.S. Dept. of HEW, Public Health Service, FDA. 5600 Fishers Lane, Rockville, Md. 20852 DHEW Publication No. (FDA) 75–4001.
Rosenblatt, Roberta. FTC Hits Midwest Ads Run by Gloria Marshall. Los Angeles Times. June 21, 1974.
Stauffer Laboratories, Inc. et al., vs. FTC. Order, Opinion, Etc., In Regard to the Alleged Violation of the FTC Act. Docket 7841. Complaint, March 21, 1960-Decision, Feb. 7, 1964.

CELLULITE

Ronsard, Nicole (Ed. Mary Butler). Cellulite. N.Y.: Beauty and Health Pub. Corp., 1973.

DIET PILLS

Diet Pill Industry. Hearings Before the Subcommittee on Antitrust and Monopoly of the Committee on the Judiciary, U.S. Senate, 90th Congress, 1968.

AMPHETAMINES

Anorectics Have No Place in the Treatment of Obesity. FDA Drug Bulletin, Dec. 1972.
Edison, George R. Amphetamines: A Dangerous Illusion. Annals of Int. Med. 74:605, 1971.

HCG

Young, R.L., et al. Chorionic Gonadotropin in Weight Control. JAMA, 236:2495, Nov. 29, 1976.

SURGERY FOR OVERWEIGHT

Study Raises Question About Ileal Bypass JAMA, 231:126, Jan. 13, 1975.

THE RICE DIET FOR EXTREME OVERWEIGHT

Kempner, W., et al. Treatment of Massive Obesity with Rice/Reduction Diet Program. Archives of Int. Med. 135:1575, Dec. 1975.

FOOD AND NUTRITION

Addis, Thomas. Glomerular Nephritis, Diagnosis and Treatment. N.Y.: Macmillan, 1952.
Boeher, L.E. Economic Aspects of Food Protein, in Sahyun, M. (Ed.), Protein and Amino Acids in Nutrition. N.Y.: Reinhold Pub. Corp., 1948.
Church, Charles F., and Church, Helen N. Food Values of Portions Commonly Used. Philadelphia: J.B. Lippincott Co., 1972.
Hegsted, et al. Protein Requirements of Adults. J. Lab. and Clin. Med. 36:261, 1946.
Research and appraisal on the "Effect of Refined Sugar and Dietary Fiber in Health and Disease," being conducted by K.K. Kimura, Medical Consultant, Life Sciences Research Office of the Federation of American Societies for Experimental Biology, 9650 Rockville Pike, Bethesda, Md. 20014
Slonaker, J.R. Stanford Univ. Press: Biological Sciences, 1939.
Watt, Bernice K., and Merrill, Annabel L. Composition of Foods: Raw, Processed and Prepared. Agriculture Handbook No. 8. U.S. Dept. of Agriculture, Washington, D.C. Reprinted, Oct. 1975.

SPECIFIC DYNAMIC ACTION OF PROTEIN NO LONGER ACCEPTED

Fletcher, Dean C., director, Section on Food Science, American Medical Assoc. Personal communication, June 3, 1976.
Miller, D.S., and Mumford, P. Obesity: Physical Activity and Nutrition. Proc. of the Nutr. Soc. (London), 25:100, 1966.

HELPFUL BOOKLETS:

Making Cheese at Home, Government Printing Office, Washington, D.C. 20402 (Describes easy method for making cottage cheese from skim milk or powdered nonfat milk).
Soybeans in Family Meals, U.S. Dept. of Agriculture Home and Garden Bulletin No. 208. (Gives a large variety of ways to use this high-protein plant food, however, the amount of fat in these recipes is unnecessarily high. I suggest cutting the amounts to one-fourth or less than the amounts given.)

OVEREATERS ANONYMOUS:

Overeaters Anonymous, World Headquarters: 2190 190th St., Torrance, Calif. 90504

INDEX

University of Southern California, 33
Ursus americanus, 27–28

vacationing, weight gain and, 10
vanity, 60, 61
vegetable(s)
  cooked
    calorie value of, 146
    cocktail, 170
    for dinner, 167, 175–177
    goulash, 176
    green beans with cream, 172
    kale and rice, 177
    kebabs, 175
    methods of cooking, 160–163
    peas and yam, 175
    spinach and bulgar, 176–177
    zucchini, chicken-stuffed, 173
  dehydrated, 163
  raw, 65, 76
    calorie value of, 144
    high in vitamin content, 210–213
    low- and very low-density, 205
    minerals in skin of, 151–152
    protein in, 144, 159
    root, 151, 152, 162
    salad, mixed, 173
  snacks, 63, 134, 179–180
  see also salads
vegetable oil, nonstick, 160
vegetarian diets, 145
vending machines, 62, 66
vinegar, 124, 164, 181
visual imagery, 75
vitamin A, 159, 210
vitamin B complex, 147, 159, 211–212
vitamin B$_{12}$, 124, 142, 143, 145, 151, 159
vitamin C, 159, 213
vitamin D, 159, 210
vitamin E, 159, 213

vitamin K, 159, 213
vitamins, 145, 151, 159
  deficiencies, 147
  dehydration and, 163
  foods high in, 210–213
vomiting, 56

walking, 57, 101
water, 62, 64, 77, 156
  see also body water
watermelon, 163
Weighing Game (Riccio and Riccio), 91
weight-control industry, 116–123
  advertising and pricing deceptions, 116–117, 118, 120, 122
weight-loss programs, *see* diet(s) and dieting; losing weight
Weight Watchers diet, 108
wheat, 146–147, 159
wine, 164, 181
Wise Woman's Diet (Christakis), 108
wok cooking, 162
Workingman's Diet, 107
working two jobs and weight gain, 9–10
writing down
  diary of food, exercise and eating, 66, 67–74, 78, 135
  reasons for weight loss, 60–61, 65

yam and peas, 175
yoga, 66
yogurt, 142, 144
You Can Do It (Proxmire), 108
"yo-yo syndrome," 85, 123, 133

Zen, 66
zinc, 151, 152
zucchini, chicken-stuffed, 173